J.-J. Merland J. Chiras

Arteriography of the Pelvis

Diagnostic and Therapeutic Procedures

With Collaboration of
M.-C. Riche J. Thiebot J.-M. Tubiana

Translated by P. Grubbe

With 105 Figures

Springer-Verlag
Berlin Heidelberg New York 1981

Authors

Professor Agr. JEAN-JACQUES MERLAND
Hôpital Lariboisière, Département de Neuroradiologie,
2, Rue Ambroise-Paré, F-75010 Paris

Dr. JACQUES CHIRAS
Chef de Clinique, Assistant des Hôpitaux,
Neuroradiologie Charcot, Hôpital de la Salpétrière,
47, Boulevard de l'Hôpital, F-75013 Paris

Collaborators

Dr. MARIE-CLAIRE RICHE
Chef de Clinique, Assistante des Hôpitaux,
Département de Radiologie, Hôpital Lariboisière,
2, Rue Ambroise-Paré, F-75010 Paris

JACQUES THIEBOT
Radiologiste des Hôpitaux, Hôpital Charles Nicolle,
C.H.R. de Rouen, F-76000 Rouen

Dr. JEAN-MICHEL TUBIANA
Chef de Clinique, Assistant des Hôpitaux,
Département de Radiologie, Hôpital Saint-Antoine,
F-75012 Paris

ISBN 3-540-10766-5 Springer-Verlag Berlin Heidelberg New York
ISBN 0-387-10766-5 Springer-Verlag New York Heidelberg Berlin

Library of Congress Cataloging in Publication Data. Merland, J.-J. (Jean-Jacques), 1942– Arteriography of the pelvis. Bibliography: p. Includes index. 1. Pelvis-Blood-vessels-Radiography. 2. Arteries-Radiography. I. Chiras, J. (Jean), 1949– . II. Title. (DNLM: 1. Embolization, Therapeutic. 2. Pelvis-Blood supply. 3. Pelvis-Radiography. 4. Angiography. WE 750 M568a) RC946.M47 616.1′307572 81-9097 AACR2

Typesetting, printing, and binding: Universitätsdruckerei H. Stürtz AG, Würzburg
2121/3140-543210

To our wives

Preface

The anatomic structure of the vascular supply of the pelvis has long been the subject of study. Progress in angiography rendered it a valuable diagnostic aid. Nevertheless, angiography is finding new applications in combination with the technique of superselective catheterization, opening the way for interventional angiography. Remarkable as this may prove, one must not overlook the difficulties involved, most of which essentially result from insufficient knowledge of the anatomic structure concerned: the pelvic arteries are particularly problematic owing to their complexity and multiple variations. For this reason we here attempt to chart precisely the course of each artery supplying the pelvis and to provide a synthetic study of the different vascular territories. The book is completed by some pathologic examples which illustrate the sometimes very important role of embolization in therapy.

Acknowledgements

This work has been produced in close collaboration with urologists, gynecologists, orthopedic surgeons, gastroitestinal surgeons, and neurosurgeons. We would particularly like to thank all those who have referred their patients to us, and especially Prof. KUSS from the Department of Urology, Hôpital La Pitie, whose role in the realization of this book was crucial, and his colleagues, Prof. LE GUILLOU, Prof. JARDIN, and Prof. CHATELAIN. Others to whom we owe our thanks in the above respect are Prof. STEG and Prof. BOCCON-GIBOD (Department of Urology, Hôpital Cochin); Prof. DUFOUR, Prof. CUKIER, and Dr. LEPAGE (Department of Urology, Hôpital Necker); Prof. MOULONGUET (Hôpital Bichat); Prof. ROY-CAMILLE and Prof. SAILLANT (Department of Orthopedics, Hôpital La Pitie); Prof. CABROL and Prof. GRANDCHBACH (Department of Cardiovascular Surgery, Hôpital La Pitie); Prof. ANDREASSIAN, (Hôpital Beaujon); Dr. GUILMET and Dr. LAURIAN (Hôpital Foch); Dr. VERGES (Hôpital Gouin); Prof. CROSNIER and Prof. KREISS; Prof. VIARS and Prof. GLASER (Department of Anesthsiology, Hôpital La Pitie); Prof. BRISSET and Prof. BOURQUELOT (Department of Urology, Hôpital St-Joseph); Prof. NATALI, Prof. KIEFFER, and Dr. TRICOT (Department of Vascular Surgery, Hôpital La Salpétrière); Prof. MERCADIER, Prof. CHIGOT, and Prof. CLOT (Department of Gastrointestinal Surgery, Hôpital La Pitie); and Dr. KORDT (Stavenger, Norway).

We also wish to thank those who have helped us in the elaboration of this work: T. LEPAGE, J.M. TUBIANA, Ph. GRENIER, T. GAVEAU, and our chief expert in radiology, Prof. J. BORIES.

Finally, we would like to express our gratitude to our colleagues from the departments of neuroradiology at Hôpital La Salpétrière and Hôpital Lariboisière, and especially to Mrs. GIRAC and Mrs. ARRAYET.

Contents

1 Technique

Almost always, routine injection of the abdominal aorta yields excellent opacification of the arteries supplying the pelvic area. In general, the results obtained are quite adequate to render selective angiography of the common iliac artery or of the trunk of the hypogastric artery unnecessary. Selective angiography is indicated, however, when various radiographic projections are to be used in the study of a specific region of the pelvis.

A. Selective Arteriography of the Hypogastric Artery

Selective arteriography of the hypogastric artery is usually carried out via the femoral approach:

1. Homolaterally, by using a sharply curved catheter or a Simmons type catheter (1, 2 or 3).
2. Contralaterally, by three different possible techniques:
   a) A long Simmons type catheter (3).
   b) A flexible catheter the tip of which is passed up into the common iliac artery from where it is slowly drawn back down and into the hypogastric artery by using a guide wire.
   c) Coaxial catheters (e.g. 7 F and 5 F): the external tube hugs the aortic bifurcation while the inner tube passes down into the hypogastric artery.

The axillary approach is only used under rare circumstances.

B. Superselective Arteriography of the Hypogastric Artery

This technique is only indicated for specific reasons: diagnostic (e.g., impotence) and above all therapeutic. Three different approaches are possible.

I. Axillary-Brachial Approach (Usually Left Side)

The puncture is made in either the axillary or brachial artery. A thin catheter (4 or 5 F) is used. This approach provides the best possible conditions for the study of the branches of the lumbar segment of the aorta as well as those of the internal and external iliac arteries. The operator can work further away from the field of irradiation. There are, however, certain risks and problems which may be encountered in this approach:

1. Spasm of the punctured artery. The chances of this occurring are lessened by using a minimally traumatic procedure combined with the use of local vasodilators and anesthetics or even heparin administration (0.5 mg/kg).
2. Risk of inserting the catheter into the orifice of the vertebral artery. This should be avoided by following the catheter by fluoroscopy.
3. Difficulty in inserting the catheter into the descending segment of the aorta when the aorta itself is slightly more enlarged than normal. In such cases a guide wire or a catheter having a larger curvature is used.

For these reasons, we often prefer to use the femoral approach.

II. Femoral Approach, Homolaterally and Contralaterally

The use of a thin-walled catheter (5 F) having a Simmons type curvature often permits a selective then superselective catheterization of the branches of the hypogastric artery, from either the homolateral or contralateral side.
Sometimes a bilateral approach is necessary. It should be noted that, when used homolaterally, the distal segment of a Simmons type catheter permits catheterization of the anterior trunk and the lateral sacral arteries, while when used contralaterally it readily catheterizes the posterior trunk. According to the indications (anterior or posterior trunk) a crossed type catheterization can be used.
The procedure using coaxial catheters can also be employed.
As a rule, the approach that is to be used is determined by the arterial conditions of the patient: for the young patient, the axillary or femoral approach; for the elderly patient, the femoral approach. In emergency situations (to achieve hemostasis by embolization), both means of approach can be used one after the other or in concert.

C. Branches of the Aorta

The lower lumbar arteries and the middle sacral artery are nowadays easily catheterized via a femoral approach according to the procedure which we have just described, using a thin-walled Simmons type catheter.
The inferior mesenteric artery, and more precisely the hemorrhoidal arteries, are more easily catheterized by means of an axillary approach. Occasionally they can be reached by using a thin-walled Simmons type catheter introduced into the femoral artery.

D. Branches of the Iliofemoral Artery

As a general rule, branches of the iliofemoral artery are accessible only to catheters which follow the direction of the blood flow, i.e., by an axillary or contralateral femoral approach. For the latter, the bifurcation of the aorta may pose some problems, so a coaxial catheter is recommended. Only the deep circumflex iliac artery can sometimes be catheterized by means of a homolateral femoral approach.

E. Patient Preparation and Surveillance During and After the Examination

Because selective and superselective angiography and embolization are usually lengthy procedures it is preferable to carry them out under either general anesthesia or neuroleptanesthesia. Catheterization of the bladder is often necessary to eliminate its opacification. Apnea as well as antispasmodics enhance radiographic substraction.
As far as laboratory tests are concerned, renal function tests as well as electrolyte levels are always necessary. These, along with diuresis, would have to be monitored during and after the examination in cases where large quantities of contrast medium are used.

F. Additional Procedures

According to the situation, it may be necessary to employ marking of the anus or urethra, rectal insufflation, opacification or insufflation of the bladder, or even uterine opacification.

G. Irradiation Protection

Pelvic exploration entails the problem of irradiation of the gonads. It is therefore necessary to assure them of a maximum amount of protection before carrying out the procedure, as well as reducing irradiation to a minimum (by using localized fields, lead pads, and adjusted equipment).
The operator should be protected by suitable screening, especially when using the femoral approach.

H. Side Effects and Accidents

We have already mentioned the technical problems which are inherent to the axillary-brachial approach, and its risks with respect to the vertebral artery.
Arterial spasm is a possibility when superselective catheterization is performed. Other clinical manifestations which may develop, above all in elderly patients or those having undergone pelvic radiation therapy, include lesions of the intima, thromboses, arterial rupture, or false aneurysms. These risks, although rare, should not be neglected because of the frequency of these types of patients in cases where embolization is indicated. In 150 arteriographic explorations of the pelvis, we observed two cases of parietal dissection without any repercussions and one case of atherosclerotic arterial fracture (the iliolumbar artery) which resulted in a retroperitoneal hematoma.

I. Embolization

I. Materials Used

Although materials used have become considerably diverse they can be grouped into three general categories:

1. Hemostatic emboli (autologous clots, Gelfoam).
2. Solid non-reabsorbable emboli (dura mater, beads, Ivalon, coils, inflatable balloons).
3. Polymerizing fluid emboli (isobutyl-2-cyano-acrylate, silicone).

II. Procedure and Choice of Material

Both depend upon what the embolization is indicated for:

1. Hemostatic embolization can be achieved by a more or less selective technique using clots or gelfoam.
2. Preoperative embolization requires solid emboli which penetrate the lesion.
3. Isolated embolization makes use of solid or liquid emboli which are determined by the particular situation. The embolization should be located as distally as possible.

III. Precautions

Wherever it is to be employed, embolization requires certain precautionary measures:

1. A complete angiographic workup of the areas to be embolized.
2. An evaluation of any possible risks of embolization to a particular area:
   a) Cutaneous, mucosal (particularly rectal), and neuronal territories.
   b) The presence of large anastomoses with other areas that may be providing a functional collateral system (the inferior gluteal and to a lesser extent the obturator arteries largely anastomosed with branches of the femoral artery).
3. A selective and stable catheterization along with a free flow injections, and the absence of any backflow.
4. Adaptation of the diameter of emboli to the shunts
5. Regular monitoring, both radiographic and fluoroscopic, should be used in order to follow the steps in the obliteration and to avoid embolization by backflow of any neighboring areas.
6. Embolization should usually begin with the major pedicles and then proceed to the accessory ones.
7. When liquid emboli (silicone, IBC) are used, coaxial catheters (e.g., 5 F and 3 F)

are a requisite. This precaution avoids any problems which may be encountered during the removal of the embolizing catheter.

IV. Side Effects

The usual side effects of embolization are:

a) Local pain, which may result in a desire to urinate in cases of embolization of the bladder, tenesmus, or desire to defecate in cases of rectal embolization.
b) Slight fever which lasts 1–2 days.
c) Electrolytic disturbances and alterations of renal function in cases where large quantities of contrast medium were used.

V. Accidental Manifestations

Such manifestations are generally due to ischemia, which may be either local or at a distance.

a) Muscular necrosis, particularly in cases of extensive bilateral and simultaneous embolization of the muscular branches of both hypogastric arteries or of the branches associated with the lumbar arteries.
b) Cutaneous and mucosal (above all rectal mucosal) necroses, which carry the risk of perforation or formation of local abcesses.
c) Neurologic disturbances, sacral or sciatic.
d) Ectopic emboli by backflow or via collateral pathways which may provoke extensive thromboses, particularly in the lower limb.

These accidents, which are quite uncommon, are more likely to occur when liquid emboli are used. In addition, when IBC is used, it may polymerize on contact with the catheter, thus rendering the removal of the catheter impossible or, if removal is possible, there is a risk of further embolization of other areas. For this reason, a very careful procedure must be followed: free flow injection, coaxial catheters, and immediate removal of the catheter after injection of a liquid embolus.

2 Normal Angiography

A. Generalities

The pelvis and its walls have an extensive vascular supply originating from three distinct sources:

1. Hypogastric system
2. Aortic system
3. Iliofemoral system

Each of its areas or organs is usually supplied by one or two of these major sources. It must be pointed out, however, that a considerable anastomotic network, which has been well documented for many years by anatomic studies, is also present.
For these reasons, we shall first present a branch-by-branch study of its arterial sources, which will be followed by a global analysis of its vascular territories.

B. Hypogastric Artery

I. Introduction

The hypogastric artery is the medial branch of the bifurcation of the common iliac artery. The hypogastric artery supplies the pelvic viscera, the pelvic walls, the gluteal and obturator regions, and under certain circumstances it provides an alternative pathway to the vascularization of the lower limb.
The branching of the hypogastric artery is subject to great variation. While some branches originate directly from the artery, many arise indirectly via a common trunk.

II. Embryology

During fetal life the pelvis and lower extremity are supplied by the branches of the umbilical artery.
During the first 3 months, the ischiatic artery, which accompanies the sciatic nerve, supplies the entire lower limb bud (Dubreuil-Chambardel 1925). Then the femoral artery, accompanying the femoral nerve, progressively extends itself to achieve, at birth, the adult disposition; this embryologic disposition explains certain vascular abnormalities encountered in the lower limb (Fig. 1) (Finerty 1949).
Following birth, the umbilical artery undergoes a certain degree of atrophy to become, on a functional level, a branch of the hypogastric artery.

III. Radiologic Anatomy

1. Origin

The hypogastric artery arises from the medial side of the common iliac artery, most frequently at the level of superior limit of the sacral wing (60% of cases); however, it may arise opposite the inferior limit of L-5 (20%) or at the level of the conjugate diameter (20%) (Fig. 2). The level of its origin descends with age. There are no notable differences between the sexes.
The angle of bifurcation, which in young subjects is quite closed, widens with age, especially when the common iliac arteries are tortuous. These alterations account for the posterior rotation of the arterial ostium, a phenomenon frequently observed in elderly patients (Fig. 3).

2. Course

The hypogastric artery extends downward, forming an anteriorly convex curve in front of the anterior surface of the sacral wing. The degree of curvature is variable, as is the length of the artery, which is usually 2–4 cm long. As a rule, the higher the origin, the longer the artery, with extreme limits of length being between 1 and 8 cm.

3. Termination

The hypogastric artery terminates at the superior limit of the greater sciatic notch by dividing into two trunks, one anterior, the other posterior (in 80% of cases), and in 20% of cases it terminates in a cluster of branches (Fig. 4). Four main branches constitute these trunks. These are the superior and inferior gluteal arteries, the obturator artery, and the inferior pudendal artery, while the other branches due to their similarities in caliber and course can be considered as branches of the four above-mentioned arteries.
The composition of the trunks can vary (Fig. 5): the superior gluteal artery is invariably the principal terminal branch of the posterior trunk (Fig. 6); the internal pudendal artery is always a terminal branch of the anterior trunk; the inferior gluteal and obturator arteries arise most often from the anterior trunk (Fig. 7), but sometimes from the posterior trunk or from its collateral branches (Fig. 30). On occasion, the obturator artery, seemingly absent, arises from a branch of the external iliac artery (Fig. 8).
The manner in which the anterior trunk terminates is also variable. It terminates either in trifurcation of the three principal branches or in a grouping off of the branches, i.e. the inferior gluteal artery and a common trunk for the obturator and internal pudendal arteries, or the obturator artery and a common trunk for the inferior gluteal and internal pudendal arteries (Fig. 9).

a) Posterior Trunk of the Hypogastric Artery

In nearly all cases it gives rise to the iliolumbar, the superior gluteal, and the lateral sacral arteries.

α) Iliolumbar Artery (Figs. 11–15)

The radiologic characteristics of the iliolumbar artery are:
a) It is the first branch of either posterior trunk or the hypogastric artery.
b) It runs upward facing the iliac wing, lateral to the hypogastric artery.
c) It divides into lateral and ascending branches at the level of L-5.

An artery of small caliber (1–2 mm), it is the first branch of the hypogastric artery. Its site of origin is, however, variable. These variations are summarized in Fig. 10. It can arise independently, or by way of a common trunk with the superior lateral sacral artery (in 12% of the cases according to DUBREUIL-CHAMBARDEL 1925, Fig. 12); it may arise from the posteriosuperior side of the posterior trunk, or in rare cases directly from the hypogastric artery. It runs upward, first crossing the external iliac vessels and then the anterior surface of the psoas muscle (Fig. 11).
The iliolumbar artery divides into two branches:

a) The iliac branch, which passes laterally, perforates the iliacus muscle, and ramifies in the iliac fossa between that muscle and the iliac bone, where it supplies a nutrient artery to the bone. Radiologically, this branch shows anastomoses with the deep circumflex iliac artery, which arises from the external iliac artery (Fig. 13). As described by anatomists, the external iliac artery runs along the iliac crest and is merely one of its anastomoses.
b) The lumbar branch has an upward lateral backward course (Fig. 14). Short in length, it supplies the psoas muscle, the quadratus lumborum muscle, and the deep spinal muscles, in addition to an area of the spine and spinal canal equivalent to a fifth lum-

bar artery. It forms anastomoses with the ipsilateral branches of the fourth lumbar and superior lateral sacral arteries. The lumbar branch may arise independently from the hypogastric artery above the iliac branch, or it may be absent, in which case it is replaced by a fifth lumbar artery (Fig. 15).

β) **Lateral Sacral Arteries** (Figs. 15–22)

These arteries constitute the second group of branches of the posterior trunk; variations in their origin are quite frequent (Fig. 16).
Although their number may vary between one and four (Fig. 17), they are classically described as being two, the superior and inferior lateral sacral arteries. They may arise independently (Fig. 19) or by a common trunk (Fig. 18) from the posteromedial side of the superior gluteal artery, from the posterior trunk, less frequently, or from the hypogastric artery (Fig. 20), and even less often from the anterior trunk (Fig. 21).
The superior lateral sacral artery may arise from a common trunk with the iliolumbar artery.
On an anteroposterior film the lateral sacral arteries are easily recognized by their lateral course toward the anterior sacral foramina.

Superior Lateral Sacral Artery (Fig. 18)

The radiologic characteristics of the superior lateral sacral artery are that it takes a medial course toward the first anterior sacral foramen, in front of which it bends at a right angle and continues upward.

It runs laterally to the first anterior sacral foramen, through which it passes and divides within the vertebral canal into two terminal branches:

a) The spinal branch, which has an upward lateral course: it forms an anastomosis with the radicular branches of the cauda equina.
b) The dorsal branch: it passes through the first posterior sacral foramen and supplies the paravertebral muscles.
c) Other branches: just before entering the anterior sacral foramen the superior lateral sacral artery gives off a presacral descending branch which anastomoses with the ipsilateral inferior lateral sacral artery. Via its muscular branches it anastomoses with the lumbar branch of the iliolumbar artery (Fig. 22).

Inferior Lateral Sacral Artery (Figs. 18, 19)

The radiologic characteristics of the inferior lateral sacral artery are:
An initial lateral course followed by bifurcation in front of the second anterior sacral foramen, giving an ascending branch and a descending branch which extends to the tip of the coccyx; and usually bilateral injection via anastomoses.

The inferior lateral sacral artery follows a lateral course toward the second anterior sacral foramen, opposite which, according to anatomists, it bends downward at a 90° angle and descends in front of the anterior sacral foramina. It terminates on the anterior surface of the coccyx by anastomosing in front of that bone with the middle sacral artery and with the inferior lateral sacral artery of the opposite side (Fig. 19).
The branches of the inferior lateral sacral artery are:

1. An ascending branch which anastomoses with the superior lateral sacral artery of the same side. Its frequently large caliber permits it to be considered radiologically as a terminal branch of the inferior lateral sacral artery.
2. Presacral branches which arise in front of each anterior sacral foramen and anastomose with the middle sacral artery.
3. Spinal branches which enter the spinal canal at the level of each anterior sacral foramen, sometimes distinguishable radiologically but as a rule only for a short distance.
4. Muscular branches feeding the piriform, greatest gluteal, levator ani, and iliococcygeal muscles. Occasionally it may supply part of the territory fed by the inferior glu-

teal artery, thus creating a rare ischiosacral trunk (Dubreuil-Chambardel 1925) (Fig. 19).

Finally, it is necessary to emphasize its extensive anastomotic networks, which in most cases allow injection into the middle sacral artery and the lateral sacral arteries on the opposite side. It invariably anastomoses with other branches of the hypogastric (the iliolumbar artery; the inferior gluteal artery via the muscular branches feeding the piriform muscle; the internal pudendal artery via its perianal branches; the obturator artery by way of its muscular branches) and other arteries, namely the middle sacral and the last lumbar arteries.

γ) Superior Gluteal Artery

The radiologic characteristics of the superior gluteal artery are that it has a large caliber, an archlike shape, extends laterally, and ramifies into multiple branches opposite the iliac wing.

The largest branch of the hypogastric artery, it almost invariably forms the terminal branch of the posterior trunk, whereas the iliolumbar and lateral sacral arteries, by their smaller caliber and their different possible origins, appear to be mere branches and not terminal branches of the posterior trunk.

Anatomically, the superior gluteal artery forms an upwardly and posteriorly concave curve under the inferior edge of the iliac wing and leaves the pelvis via the great sciatic foramen above the piriform muscle (Figs. 23, 24).
In the gluteal region, it divides into two terminal branches:

a) The superficial branch (Figs. 25, 26) passes upward and laterally between the greatest and middle gluteal muscles, assuring their blood supply as well as the skin which cover them.
b) The deep branch (Fig. 27) runs laterally, passing between the middle and least gluteal muscles, which it supplies.

In its intrapelvic course the superior gluteal artery gives off anastomotic branches to the lateral sacral, the iliolumbar, and the inferior gluteal arteries as well as to the branches of the iliofemoral axis.

Radiologically (Fig. 23), its trunk is easily recognizable by its large caliber and its lateral course, which forms an upwardly and posteriorly concave curve that crosses the hip bone. It divides into two branches: the deep branch, which is largest, following the course of the superior gluteal trunk and dividing into two principal branches which are relatively constant. The first branch runs laterally, the second passes upward and laterally. This latter branch has often been mistaken for the superficial branch. As for the superficial branch itself, which is often thinner, its identification is made by applying anatomic facts (Figs. 25–27). It arises immediately after passing through the great sciatic foramen, at which point it becomes superficial. Its initial segment, which runs in an anteroposterior direction, shows up on an arteriograph viewed in the same direction as a bow-shaped image. It then ramifies into multiple branches which follow a lateral upward course. It should be pointed out that the superior gluteal artery may form a common trunk with the inferior gluteal artery (20%–30% of the cases) or may give off the obturator artery.

b) Anterior Trunk

The anterior trunk is not as well defined as the posterior trunk, as was revealed previously during study of the termination of the hypogastric artery.
The parietal branches usually number three (the inferior gluteal, the obturator, and the internal pudendal). The radiologic projections of their courses in the pelvic cavity are similar (Fig. 28), and differentiation is only possible if bony landmarks are established or the opacified territories identified. All of the visceral branches (vesical, genital, middle hemorrhoidal arteries), arise from the anterior trunk or from one of its branches (in this case almost always from the internal pudendal). Their ori-

gins, however, are not always easily identified without hyperselective injection.

α) Parietal Branches

Inferior Gluteal Artery (Figs. 28–32)

The radiologic characteristics of the inferior gluteal artery are:

a) Variable intrapelvic course forming a semicircle which is open laterally.
b) Terminates behind the neck of the femur where it breaks up into a number of diverging branches that course in a downward lateral manner.

During embryonic life, the inferior gluteal artery supplies the inferior extremity. Gradually the femoral artery assumes this role, and at birth the inferior gluteal artery supplies the inferior portion of the buttocks and the posterior proximal part of the thigh.
Nevertheless, a few cases have been reported where the embryonic arterial disposition has been found in an adult (see Fig. 1).
The artery arises most often from the anterior trunk: however, in 20%–30% of cases, it arises from the posterior trunk or from the superior gluteal artery (Fig. 30).
In most cases it courses initially downward in front of the piriform muscle and sacral plexus; it then curves laterally and leaves the pelvic cavity via the greater sciatic foramen. In the pelvic cavity, its origin is most commonly median to the internal pudendal artery, behind which it passes in its lateral course. In 15% of cases, however, its origin is lateral to the internal pudendal artery (Fig. 29). When the inferior gluteal artery arises from the superior gluteal artery, its point of origin is at different locations after the greater sciatic foramen; in such cases it sometimes courses behind the piriform muscle (Fig. 30b). The following rare variation has been noted: duplication of the inferior gluteal artery, with the other arising from a common trunk with the lateral inferior sacral arteries. Two such cases have been reported anatomically (DUBREUIL-CHAMBARDEL 1925) and we have had two similar cases (Fig. 18).

In the gluteal region the inferior gluteal artery divides into two types of branches:

a) Posterior branches coursing horizontally or ascending toward the inferior portion of the greatest gluteal muscle and the overlying skin; they anastomose with the superficial branches of the gluteal artery.
b) Descending branches which supply the posterior part of the thigh; the semitendinous, biceps femoris, gemelli, and quadratus femoris muscles.

The sciatic nerve artery (Fig. 32) is an important branch rarely recognized on the films because of its narrow caliber and its ascending rectilinear course. These branches anastomose with the perforating arteries of the deep femoral artery and the medial circumflex artery. The frequency of narrow intrapelvic branches should be noted: they course in a medial direction and supply the piriformis muscle. These branches are frequently well visualized during arteriography (we have not found an anatomic description for these arteries) (Fig. 31).
This group of arteries appears to rise nearly always where the direction of the inferior gluteal artery changes in leaving the pelvic cavity. These arteries run medially and supply the iliococcygeal muscle. Therefore opacification of the arteries is not surprising following injection of the inferior lateral sacral artery and vice versa.

This group of arteries can be erroneously confused with visceral branches: vesical and hemorrhoidal arteries. Insufflation of the organs permits their differentiation. It should be noted that the inferior gluteal artery, by its situation alone, cannot give off visceral branches. The different descending branches of the inferior gluteal artery course downward and laterally behind the femoral head and acetabulum. These branches are characteristic of the inferior gluteal artery.

Obturator Artery (Figs. 33–35)

The radiologic characteristics of the obturator artery are that it courses along the brim of the pelvis, then bifurcates above the obturator notch into two branches which run along the course of the ischiopubic and iliopubic rami.

Its origin is extremely variable (DUBREUIL-CHAMBARDEL 1925). It usually arises from the anterior trunk (70%), occasionally from the posterior trunk or one of its branches (Fig. 34), and sometimes from the inferior epigastric artery (Fig. 35).

Its course is characteristic. It is the most lateral branch of the anterior trunk and runs downward, forming a medial concave curve slightly below the brim of the pelvis. It runs behind the iliopubic ramus, passes via the obturator canal, and terminates at the margin of the obturator foramen beneath the external obturator muscle. At this point it divides into two branches, anterior and posterior.

During its intrapelvic course it gives off muscular branches and an anastomotic branch with the iliac branch of the iliolumbar artery; a pubic branch which runs behind the pubis and anastomoses with its fellow of the opposite side (Fig. 33); and an anastomotic branch with the epigastric artery of variable functional importance. It may give off visceral branches.

The obturator artery divides into two terminal branches: the anterior branch runs around the medial margin of the obturator foramen and anastomoses with the medial circumflex artery (branch of the deep femoral). It supplies branches to the layers of the testicle as well as the obturator and adductor muscles.

The posterior branch skirts the lateral margin of the obturator foramen, supplies branches to the muscles of the obturator region, and anastomoses with the inferior gluteal artery. This branch gives off an important artery, the acetabular artery, whose territory is clearly identifiable by arteriography. The acetabular artery is clearly visible and is easily identified by its recurrent ascending course, passing under the transverse ligament into the hip joint. It supplies the ligamentum teres, but its contribution to the blood supply of the head of the femur is minimal.

Internal Pudendal Artery (Figs. 36–43)

The radiologic characteristics of the internal pudenal artery are:

a) A downward medial intrapelvic course.
b) It becomes horizontal just below the symphysis and it terminates on the midline.
c) Dense opacification at the base of the corpus bulbocavernosum.

FARABEUF (1905) considered the internal pudendal artery to be a terminal branch of the hypogastric artery. It supplies the perineum and the external genitalia.

The internal pudendal artery always arises from the anterior division of the hypogastric artery and then courses downward along the anterior surface of the piriform muscle and sacral plexus, lateral to the inferior gluteal artery. It leaves the pelvis between the piriform and coccygeal muscles and passes over the ischial spine to enter the ischiorectal fossa through the small sciatic foramen. It takes a turn, and its course becomes downward, median and anterior, running parallel to the median surface of the internal obturator muscle. It then runs forward in the ischiorectal fossa and divides into two terminal branches: the perineal artery and the artery of the penis (or clitoris) just below the midpoint of the symphysis.

On the anterior posterior films (Fig. 36) its initial course is pratically vertical, but then, after crossing the sciatic spine, it takes a medial turn from the obturator foramen. The last 2 cm course horizontally just below the symphysis until reaching the midline. During arteriography, a blush appears before the rest of the artery. This is explained by the early opacification of the root of the corpus bulbocavernosum.

1. *Collateral Branches of the Internal Pudendal Artery*. The initial segement of the internal pudendal artery occasionally gives off radiologically identifiable arteries. If so, it gives small branches to the greatest gluteal

muscle. More frequently an artery of significant caliber arises behind the sciatic spine and courses laterally. Anatomic and radiologic comparison leads us to believe that this artery divides into two branches that supply the top of the acetabulum and the gemelli muscles (Fig. 37).

In the perineal region, the internal pudendal artery gives off much larger branches:

a) The inferior rectal artery, which gives rise to three branches which run medially and downward to the anus, where they supply the fascia, skin, and the elevator ani and external sphincter muscles (Fig. 36). Arteriography of the internal pudendal artery poorly distinguishes these branches. This is improved by selective injection of the middle and superior rectal arteries, which in turn opacify the inferior rectal by their anastomoses (Fig. 56).
b) The perineal artery, which is of rather large caliber (Fig. 36) and prolongates the downward couse of the internal pudendal artery. It passes behind the transverse perineal muscle and then runs forward between the ischiocavernosus and bulbocavernosus muscles to the scrotum. The artery anastomoses with external pudendal arteries, which are branches of the femoral artery (Fig. 38).
c) The artery of the bulb, which takes a medial direction through the deep transverse muscle of perineum and the urogenital diaphragm to the bulb. The artery is short and thick and is distinguished by a blush during early opacification of the root of the corpus bulbocavernosum. In addition, the artery gives off small branches to Cowper's glands (Fig. 39) and the posterior portion of the corpus spongiosum.
d) The urethral artery: short and thin, this branch passes by the posterior surface of the posterior urethra and then into the corpus cavernosum urethral.
e) Two other very fine branches must be reported: the anterior vesical artery only visible via its anastomotic pathway and a retropubic ramus.

2. *Terminal Branches of the Internal Pudendal Artery*

a) The cavernosum artery: usually thin, it penetrates the corpus cavernosum at its posterior end and runs to the tip of the penis. It runs just above the urethra in a rectilinear (Fig. 39) fashion and is easily followed. The cavernous artery anastomoses with its fellow on the other side, as evidenced by simultaneous opacification.
b) The dorsal artery of the penis, which occasionally arises in midperineum. It ascends and perforates the suspensory ligament of the penis, then runs on the superior surface of the corpus cavernosum to the glans. The artery is best viewed when the penis is stretched laterally or by a lateral view of the urethra.

The dorsal artery of the penis ramifies into numerous branches around the glans. The artery gives off many small lateral branches near the glans and the root of the penis.

Out of all of these branches, the dorsal artery of the penis is always identifiable. It should be noted that the radiographic examination performed with the penis in a flaccid state can in no way give an accurate picture of the arteries during erection.

Thus the internal pudendal artery anastomoses with the obturator artery, external pudendal artery, middle hemorrhoidal artery, and contralateral internal pudendal artery by means of its collateral and terminal branches (Fig. 38).

In the female, the internal pudendal artery is rather thin and terminates by the labial arteries and perineal artery (Fig. 43).

In order to study the venous network of the internal pudendal veins, specific measures must be taken (ample quantity of radiopaque agent, low pressure injection, adjunction of a vasodilator). Once these measures are taken, the study of the corpus cavernosum and its communications with the pudendal plexis is possible (Figs. 41, 42).

β) Visceral Branches

The practically limitless number of different anatomic descriptions of the visceral branches is understandable given its countless variations. The regions supplied, however, remain fairly invariable (Fig. 44).
Three arterial groups can be individualized: the vesical arteries, the genital arteries, and the middle rectal artery. The vesical and genital arteries have various relations. According to FARABEUF (1905), CERF (1896), and HOVELACQUE, an umbilical-vesical artery (Fig. 44), also known as the umbilical artery, is present and gives off the superior vesical artery and genital-vesical artery, which in turn gives off a vesical-prostatic artery and vesicular deferential artery (Fig. 45).
According to GOUAZE et al. (1956), and DUCLOS (1972), there is an independent prostatic artery and an umbilical-vesical artery which supplies the entire bladder and gives off the vesicular-deferential artery (Fig. 46).

γ) Vesical Arteries (Figs. 46–50)

Umbilical Artery (Fig. 47)

The radiologic characteristics of the umbilical artery are:
a) Empty bladder: suprapubic, downward, medial course.
b) Full bladder: course typically downward and median, then takes a sharp turn. Terminates by numerous inferiorly concave branches. The superior vesical branches course along the top of the bladder.

In the fetus, the umbilical arteries are the main channels of the umbilical cord. At birth they regress and only the vesical arteries retain a functional role in the adult. The umbilical artery arises from the anterior surface of the anterior division of the hypogastric artery or from one of its branches, either singularly or by a common trunk formed with the deferential artery. It has a downward medial course until it reaches the lateral surface of the bladder, at which point it takes an upward medial course.

The umbilical artery gives off two or three superior vesical arteries which supply up to 80% of the bladder (BRAITHWAITE 1952). The relationships of these arteries depend on the fullness of the bladder (Fig. 48).
When the bladder is empty (Fig. 49) the vesical artery and its branches are located just above the pubis. They are not easily distinguished from branches leading to the internal genitalia. When the bladder is filled artificially or naturally, however, the stem of the vesical artery takes on its typical "hair pin" shape and its branches spread out over the top of the bladder; in this manner their identification is possible (Fig. 50).
These arteries anastomose with other vesical arterial pedicles, notably the inferior vesical artery, which usually arises from the genital-vesical artery, but on occasion arises from the umbilical artery.

Inferior Vesical Artery (Figs. 48–50)

The radiologic characteristics of the inferior vesical artery are:
a) A downward medial course.
b) A suprapubic position.
c) It gives off ascending branches.
d) It anastomoses with the superior vesical artery.

The inferior vesical artery can arise from the umbilical, deferential, or prostatic artery. Because of its thinness, it is difficult to individualize. It supplies the lower part of the bladder and the trigone. In contrast to the superior vesical artery, its relationships are not affected by the degree of bladder fullness.

δ) Genital Arteries in the Male (Fig. 51)

Prostatic Artery (Fig. 52)

The radiologic characteristics of the prostatic artery are:

a) A suprapubic, downward, medial course.
b) It divides at the lateral angle of the prostate into two or three branches.
c) Injection of the prostatic space during capillary filling.

The prostatic artery arises from the anterior division of the hypogastric artery or from the internal pudendal artery. The prostatic artery has a downward medial course running just above the iliopubic ramus and terminates at the lateral angle of the prostate by two branches: (a) a superior branch which courses along the superior edge of the prostate and then turns downward and which supplies the portion of the prostate in contact with the urethra; and (b) a posterolateral branch which supplies the lateral portions of the prostate.
During capillary filling, the opacified prostate lobe resembles a "horn" whose base is median and whose point is superolateral. It should be noted that because of the presence of a raphe, the other half of the prostate does not become injected.

Vesicular Deferential Artery (Figs. 46, 47). This very thin artery has a downward medial course roughly parallel to the prostatic artery. After a short course it divides into two vesicular and deferential branches:

a) The vesicular branch is characteristically tortuous and has a downward medial course. It terminates just above the midpoint of the symphysis.
b) The deferential branch: this thin artery runs toward the pelvic portion of the vas deferens. Upon contact, it makes a "T" division; the medial division is short and supplies the ejaculatory duct; the lateral division leaves the minor pelvis by the inguinal canal and then courses characteristically along the vas deferens in the spermatic cord; it anastomoses with the external spermatic artery. This branch is rarely identifiable.

ε) Internal Genital Arteries in the Female

Uterine Artery (Figs. 53–54)

The radiologic characteristics of the uterine artery are:

a) "U"-shaped course.
b) Its ascending part gives off numerous convoluted branches that ramify horizontally.
c) Configuration variable according to uterine position.
d) Dense opacification of half of the uterus.

It is the homologue in the female of the deferential artery in the male, and therefore experiences the same variations converning its origin.
The uterine artery's course is typically divided into four portions (Fig. 53):

1. A short parietal segment which runs downward and medially through the lateral pelvic corrective tissue.
2. A transversal ligament segment which courses medially across the broad ligament.
3. A segment which curves upward, thus creating the uterine arch, in contact with the supravaginal wall of the cervix. This segment is more or less coiled and tortuous according to age and functional state. At this point the artery runs in the parametrium along the side of the uterus.
4. At the superior angle of the uterus, the artery penetrates the broad ligament and runs laterally to the ovary, where the artery terminates by anastomosing with the ovarian artery.

The uterine artery gives off many branches:

1. From the arch arise the cervical and vaginal arteries which supply the fundus of the bladder.
2. During its course along the side of the uterus arise numerous short and long convoluted branches which account for the dense opacification of the corresponding half of the uterus during capillary filling.
3. The tubular branches which form an arterial arcade along the fallopian tube.

The appearance of the uterine artery changes with the position of the uterus (Fig. 54). In retroversion, the segment lateral to the uterus appears straight, whereas in anteversion it seems to course away.

Vaginal Artery (Fig. 55). In most cases the vaginal artery arises from the anterior division of the hypogastric artery just below the uterine artery, but on occasion it arises from a common trunk formed with the uterine artery or with the middle rectal artery. This artery is short and difficult to identify. It descends medially and supplies the posterior and anterior surfaces of the vagina by means of four or five small branches.

Middle Rectal (Hemorrhoidal) Artery
(Figs. 56–59)

The radiologic characteristics of the middle artery are:

a) An intrapelvic downward median course.
b) It terminates behind the midpoint of the pubis in the form of a vertical vascular network.
c) Marked opacification of the inferior portion of the rectum more clearly visible following insufflation.
d) Retrograde opacification of the superior rectal artery.

The middle rectal artery is the most posterior trunk of the anterior division of the hypogastric artery. Most often it is singular, but in 29% of cases it is double. Its origin is variable, arising alone when the hypogastric artery terminates in a cluster of branches. Often it arises from the internal pudendal or obturator arteries near their origins, and other times from a common trunk with a genitovesical artery.

The middle rectal artery descends medially to the side of the middle portion of the rectum, dividing into three or four branches that circle the anterior and posterior surfaces of the rectum and anastomose with their fellows on the opposite side. In this way a notable network is created in the submucosa which anastomoses with the superior and inferior rectal arteries. This network is usually opacified by retrograde techniques. In certain cases, this same network furnishes the entire blood supply of the rectal ampulla (Fig. 58).

The middle rectal artery often sends a few small branches to the posterior portion of the bladder, the levator ani muscle, and it anastomoses to the inferior portion of the vaginal artery in the female, and on occasion to the inferior vesical artery.

It should be noted that, with the exception of pathologic circumstances where it is dilated, the middle rectal artery is difficult to catheterize because of its narrow caliber.

C. Pelvic Branches of the Abdominal Aorta

The pelvic branches comprise the middle sacral artery, the superior rectal artery, and the spermatic or ovarian artery.

I. Radiologic Anatomy

1. Middle Sacral Artery (Figs. 60–61)

The radiologic characteristics of the middle sacral artery are:

a) Central location.
b) Vertical course along the anterior surface of the sacrum.
c) Extension to the point of the coccyx, where it anastomoses with the lateral sacral arteries.

The middle sacral artery, singular and centrally placed, represents the vestiges of the sacrococcygeal portion of the aorta. It arises 1 cm above the posterior surface of its bifurcation, in most cases directly from the aorta (Fig. 60), but on occasion from a common trunk with the fourth or fifth lumbar artery (Fig. 61). The middle sacral artery passes downward into the pelvis and terminates at the tip of the coccyx where it anastomoses with the lateral sacral arteries.

Along the course of the artery, the following parietal and visceral collateral branches arise:

a) Parietal branches: next to each anterior sacral foramen a small horizontal branch arises which anastomoses with a homologous artery that arises from the lateral sacral artery;
b) Small branches, occasionally identifiable, which supply the anterior surface of the sacrum and the periosteum;
c) Visceral branches: these branches are very thin and they anastomose with the rectal arteries. They furnish a small part of the blood supply to the rectum and provide it with a collateral system which should not be overlooked.

2. Superior Rectal Artery (Fig. 62)

The radiologic characteristics of the superior rectal artery are that:

a) It is the medial branch of the inferior mesenteric artery.
b) It bifurcates and takes on a "crab claw" shape, parallel to the rectal ampulla.
c) It exhibits concomitant opacification of the inferior and middle rectal arteries.

The superior rectal artery, which is the continued trunk of the inferior mesenteric artery, arises at the level of the second or third sacral segment. It runs downward behind the rectum then divides into two branches. One continues and supplies the posterior surface of the rectum; the other, of smaller caliber, runs to and supplies its anterior surface. These two branches form the characteristic "crab claw" image, along with a marked injection of the rectal mucosa during capillary filling.

This is more readily demonstrated when a rectal insuflation is initially performed. At the base of the rectal ampulla the branches curve medially and anastomose with branches of the middle rectal artery whose course is more vertical. They supply the anal canal. The superior rectal artery invariably gives off a branch that anastomoses with the ascending or descending branch of the sigmoid artery (Sudek's arcade).

The superior rectal artery supplies the entire rectal ampulla. In cases where it is hypoplasic, the rectum is supplied by the middle rectal artery (Fig. 58).

3. Spermatic and Ovarian Arteries (Fig. 63)

The migration of the gonads during fetal life provides an explanation for their long length and lumbar-aortic site of origin. Both arteries have analogous relations in the lumbar region.

a) Right and Left Internal Spermatic Arteries (Fig. 63)

These arteries arise from the front of the abdominal aorta at the L-2 or L-3 level between the origins of the renal and inferior mesenteric arteries. They follow a sinuous, lateral, downward course. They cross the psoas muscle, pass laterally to the ureter, and continue under the peritoneum.

In their course the spermatic veins, lymphatics, and nerves accompany the arteries. The inguinal and scrotal segments of the artery are enclosed in the spermatic cord.

The branches of the internal spermatic artery are: the epididymal arteries, which anastomose with the deferential artery (branch of the vesical artery), the external spermatic artery (branch of the epigastricarteus), and the testicular arteries.

b) Ovarian Arteries (Fig. 64)

Throughout their course ovarian veins, lymphatics, and occasionally an accessory ovarian artery accompany the ovarian arteries. They penetrate the broad ligament and bifurcate into terminal branches: one anastomoses with a branch of the uterine artery; the other, of smaller caliber, also anastomoses with the uterine artery. Their sinuous course is as characteristic as that of the spermatic arteries.

The ovarian and spermatic arteries are practically invisible during lumbar arteriography. Selective injection is useful in cases of ectopic testes in the male. In the female it is useful for cases of hypervascularized processes and tubular or uterine hemorrhage.

D. Branches of the Iliofemoral Axis

The deep circumflex iliac artery, the epigastric artery, the external pudendal artery and the psoas arteries, which arise from the iliofemoral axis, give off branches that supply the pelvic walls.

I. Radiologic Anatomy

1. Deep Circumflex Iliac Artery (Fig. 13)

The radiologic characteristics of the deep circumflex iliac artery are:

a) It arises from the lateral side of the external iliac artery just above the inguinal ligament.
b) It runs laterally toward the anterior superior spine of the ilium.

At the anterior superior spine of the ilium it divides into two terminal branches:

a) The medial branch, which supplies the psoas, iliac, sartorius, tensor fasciae latae, and the oblique and transverse muscles of the abdomen.
b) The iliac branch passes around the crest of the ilium and gives off small branches for the rectus muscles, these branches anastomose with branches of the fourth lumbar artery. It also gives off small vertical branches which supply the iliac muscle and anastomose with branches of the iliolumbar artery (Fig. 13).

2. Inferior Epigastric Artery (Figs. 25–66)

The radiologic characteristics of the inferior epigastric artery are:

a) It arises from the external iliac artery just above the inguinal ligament.
b) Its initial segment forms an inverted arch and upward medial course.

The inferior epigastric artery arises from the medial side of the external iliac artery just above the inguinal ligament; its initial segment forms an inverted arch and then continues upward and medially toward the rectus muscle and its sheath, which it penetrates.
Along its course the inferior epigastric artery gives off three important branches:

1. A branch which anastomoses with the obturator artery. Its caliber is variable and in certain cases it supplies the territory usually supplied by the obturator artery. In such cases the obturator artery arises from the epigastric arch.
2. The external spermatic artery of small caliber is usually invisible during arteriography. It joins the other elements which make up the spermatic cord and terminates in the fascia of the testicule.
3. A small suprapubic branch which runs along the superior edge of the pubis and anastomoses with its fellow of the opposite side and with a branch of the internal pudendal artery. The caliber of this anastomosis is variable. The dorsal artery of the penis can arise from the epigastric artery (Dubreuil-Chambardel 1925).

3. External Pudendal Arteries (Fig. 67)

The radiologic characteristics of the external pudendal arteries are: it arises from the femoral artery, it runs medially, and it terminates below the pubis at its midpoint.

The arteries arise from the medial side of the femoral artery by a common trunk. They run medially in the subcutaneous tissue and pass behind the ramus of the ischium. The trunk terminates near the inguinal ligament by dividing into two branches:

1. One branch supplies the tissues which cover the pubic area.
2. The other branch supplies the scrotum and perineum in the male and the labia majora in the female.

These branches anastomose with small branches of the internal pudendal artery.

4. Psoas Arteries

These arteries are invariably present but usually invisible during arteriography. They vary in number and arise at different points from the external iliac artery, either by multiple arterioles (60% of cases), or by a single trunk which runs lateral to the anterior surface of the psoas muscle. These arteries anastomose with branches of the iliolumbar and deep circumflex iliac arteries.

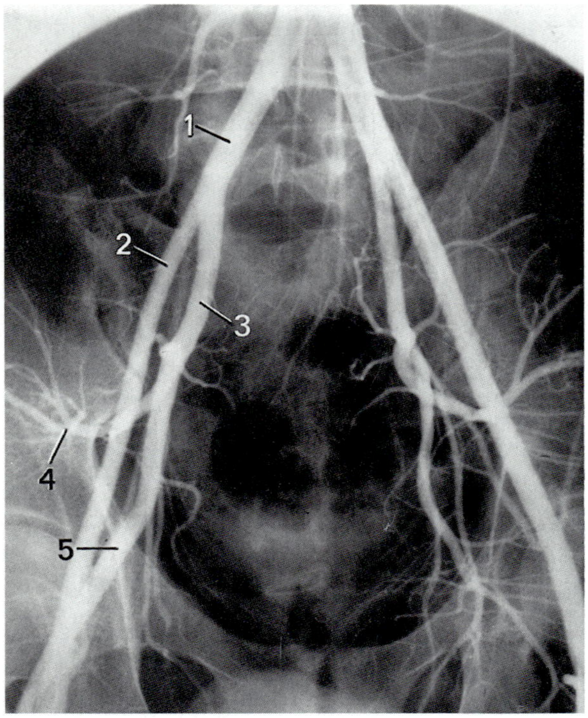

Fig. 1. Global arteriography in a 20-year-old man. There is a persistent ischiatic artery on the right side. It runs along the back side of the thigh, gives off the popliteal artery and supplies the leg. In this case the femoral artery only supplies the anterior part of the thigh
1 common iliac artery
2 external iliac artery
3 internal iliac artery
4 superior gluteal artery
5 inferior gluteal artery (or persistent ischiatic artery)

Fig. 2a–c see p. 19

Fig. 3 a, b. Because the arteries in elderly patients are more tortuous than in younger patients, the interpretation of global angiography is more difficult, as are superselective catheterizations (same legends as Fig. 2)
▽

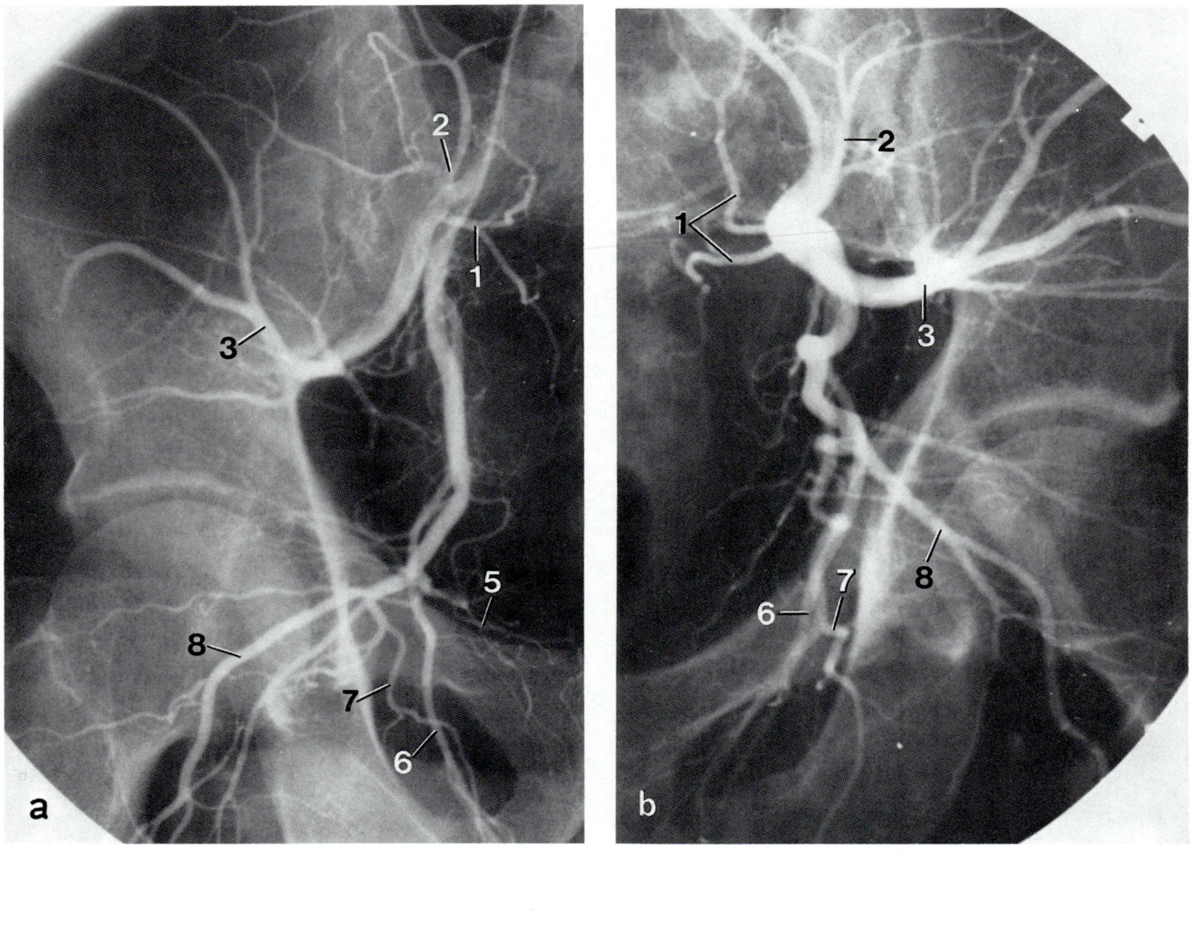

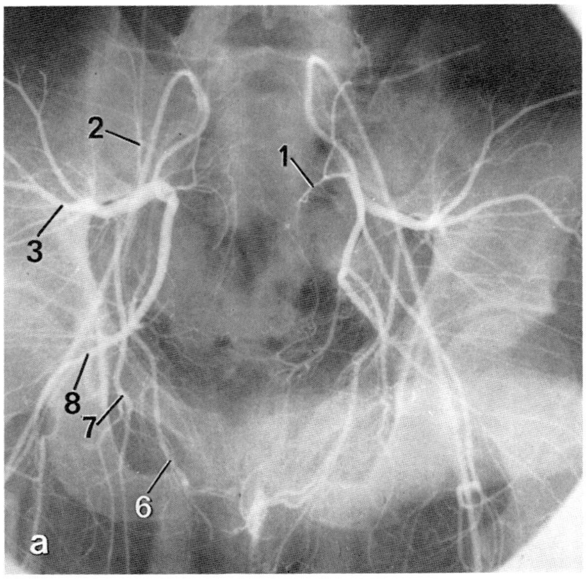

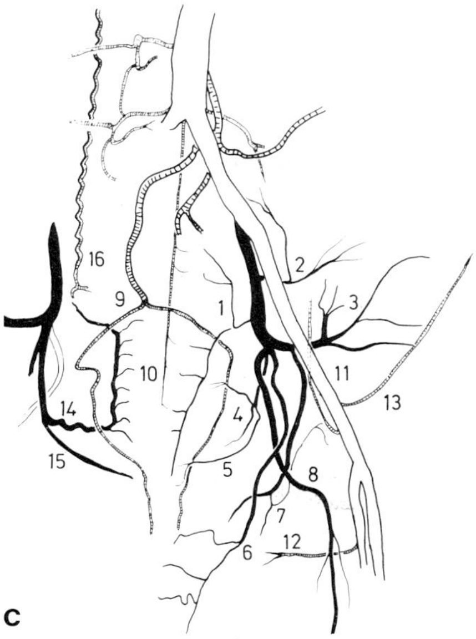

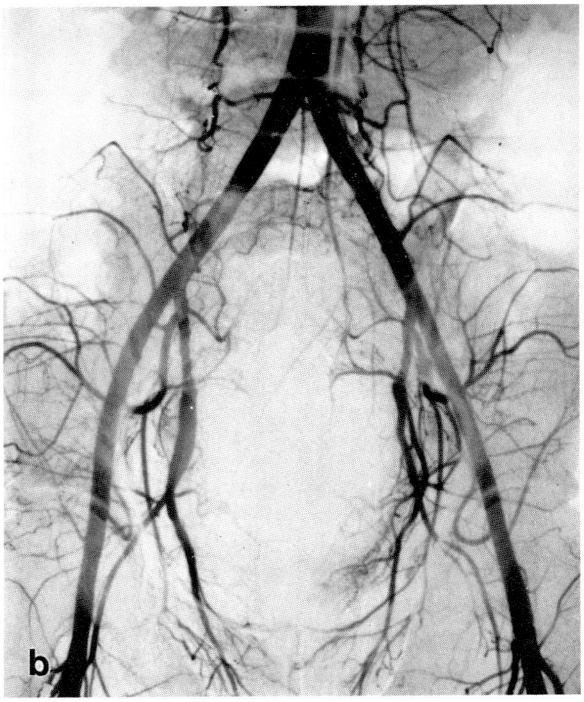

Fig. 2 a–c. Bilateral or unilateral femoral puncture gives the same results as a selective arteriography of the internal iliac artery. The internal iliac artery may arise in front of the sacral wing **a** or in front of the vertebral foramen between L-4 and L-5. **c** Schema

1 lateral sacral artery
2 iliolumbar artery
3 superior gluteal artery
4 superior vesical artery
5 inferior vesical artery
6 internal pudendal artery
7 obturator artery
8 inferior gluteal artery
9 superior hemorrhoidal artery
10 medial sacral artery
11 inferior epigastric artery
12 external pudendal artery
13 superficial iliac circumflex artery
In female:
14 uterine artery
15 vaginal artery
16 ovarian artery

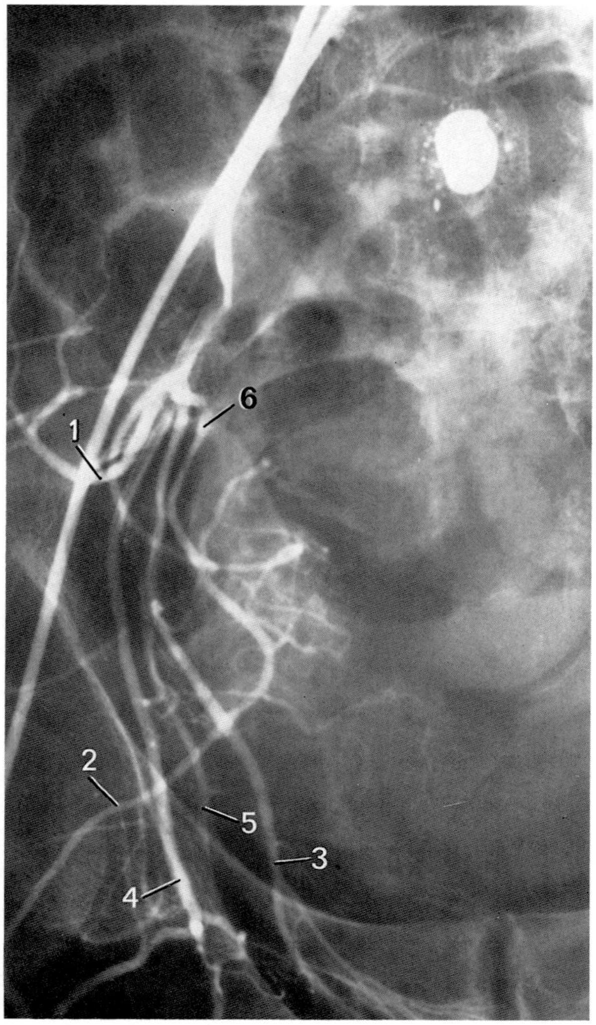

Fig. 4. Termination of the hypogastric artery in a cluster of branches
1 superior gluteal artery
2 inferior gluteal artery
3 internal pudendal artery
4 obturator artery
5 umbilical artery
6 middle rectal artery

Fig. 5 a–f. Main variations in the division of the anterior trunk. **a** Inferior gluteal (*1*), internal pudendal (*2*) and obturator (*3*) arteries (The same numbering applies to **b–f**). **b** Inferior gluteal and internal pudendal arteries. **c** Internal pudendal and obturator arteries. **d** Inferior gluteal artery arising from superior gluteal artery. **e** Obturator artery arising from superior gluteal artery. **f** Division of anterior trunk into its various branches without a common trunk ▷

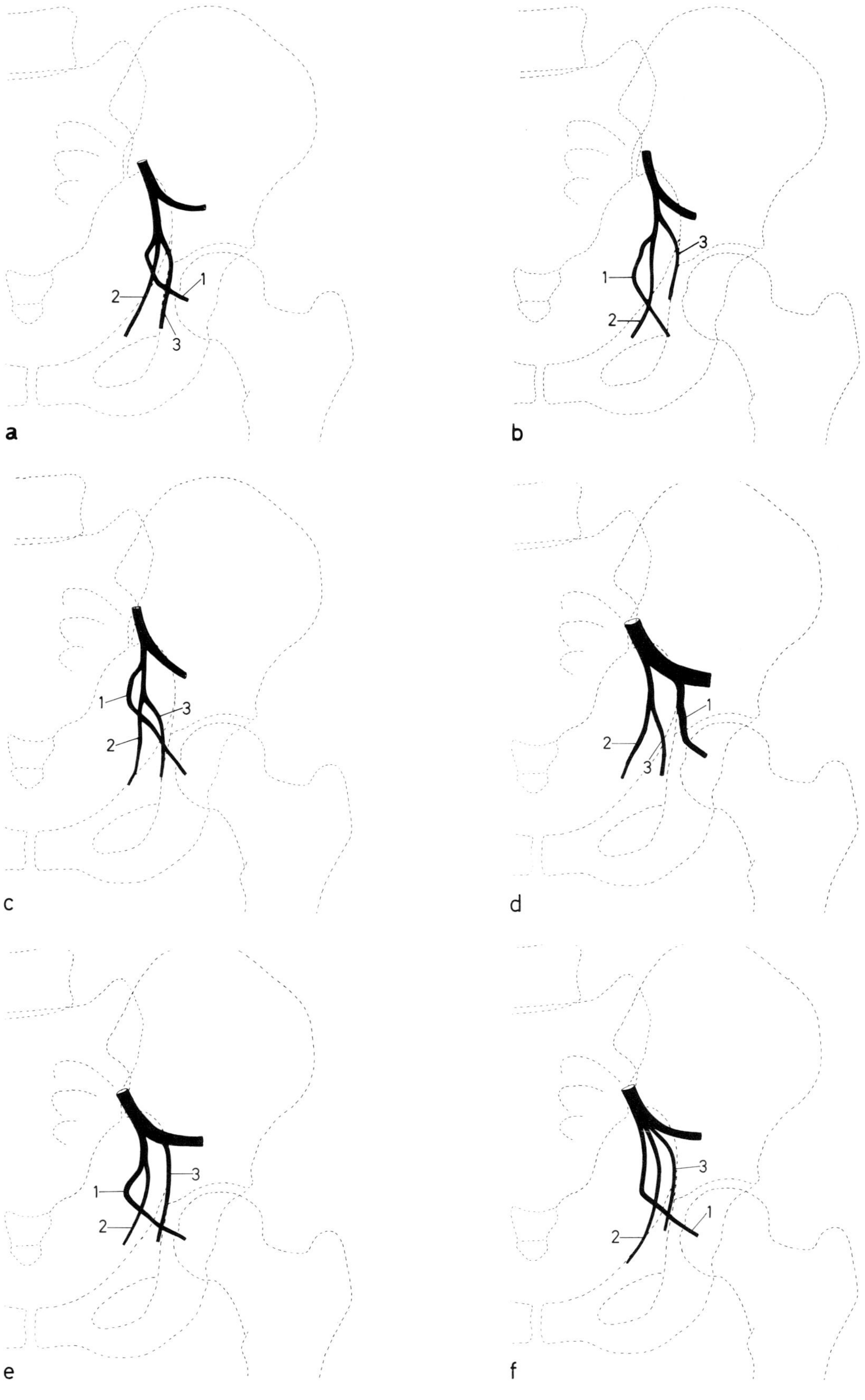
1
2
3
a
b
c
d
e
f

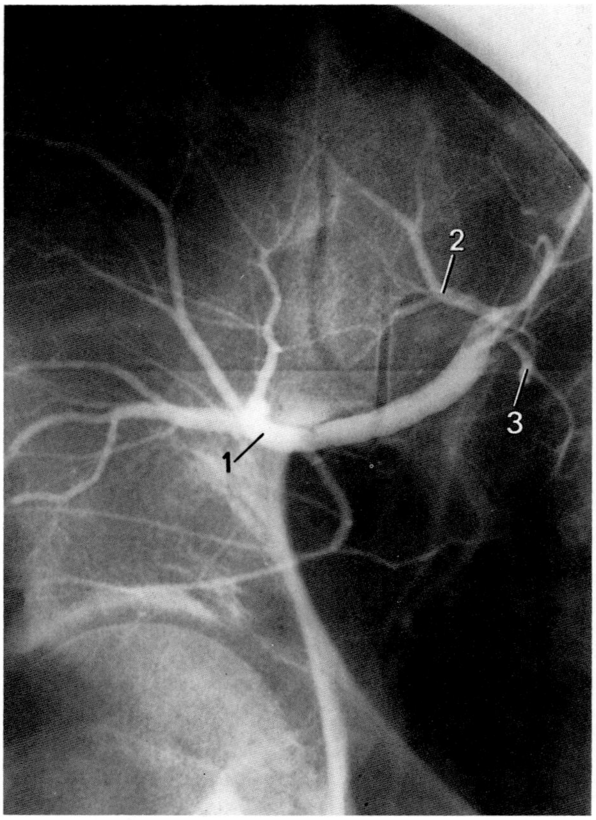

Fig. 6. Posterior trunk
1 superior gluteal artery
2 iliolumbar artery
3 lateral sacral artery

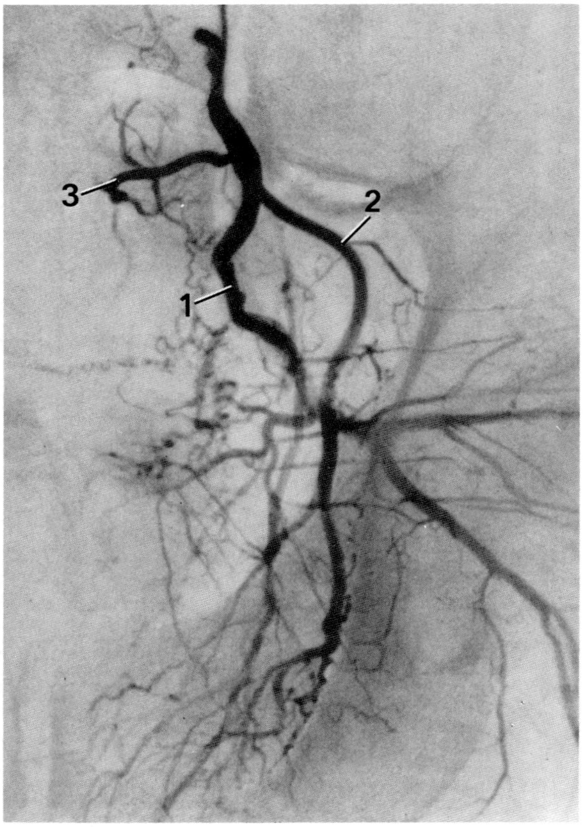

Fig. 7. Inferior gluteal artery (*1*), obturator artery (*2*) and inferior sacral lateral artery (*3*) arising from the anterior trunk of the internal iliac artery

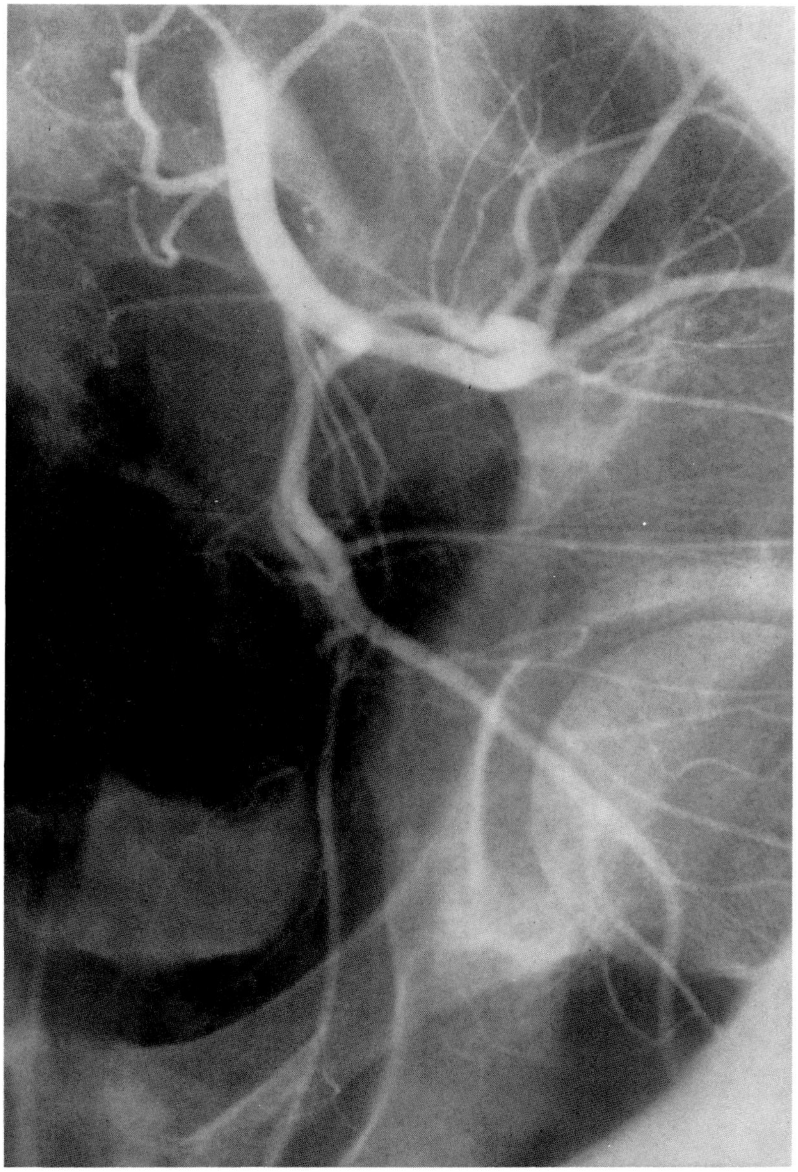

Fig. 8. In some cases the obturator artery may arise from the external iliac artery or from one of its branches, particularly the inferior epigastric artery

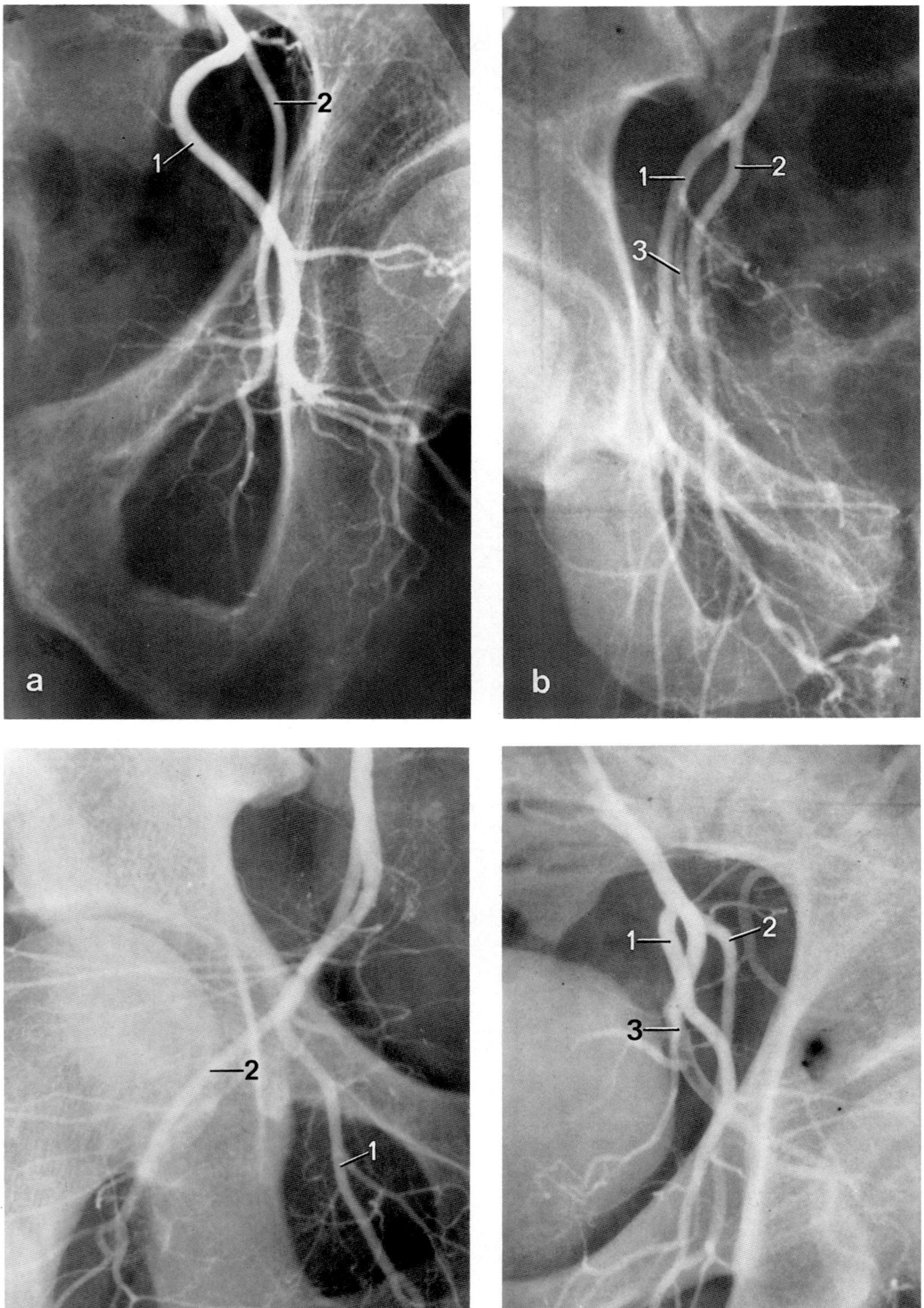
2
1
a
1
2
3
b
2
1
c
1
2
3
d

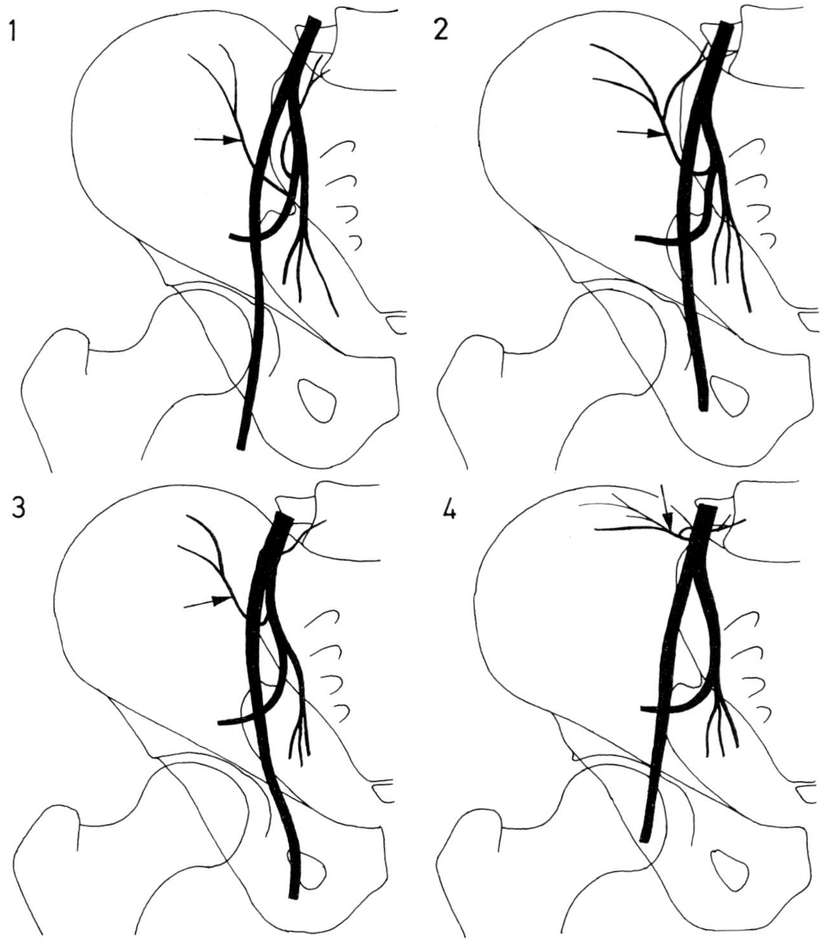

Fig. 10. Variations in the origin of the iliolumbar artery
1 separate origin of the two branches from the posterior trunk
2 common origin from the posterior trunk (most frequent variety)
3 lumbar branch arising from the common iliac artery
4 iliolumbar artery originating from the common iliac artery

◁ **Fig. 9 a–d.** Various types of anterior trunks. **a** Inferior gluteal (*1*) and obturator arteries (*2*). **b** Obturator (*1*) and internal pudendal arteries (*2*) branching off genitovesical artery (*3*). **c** Inferior gluteal (*2*) and internal pudendal arteries (*1*). **d** Division in three main branches: internal pudendal artery (*1*), obturator artery (*2*), and inferior gluteal artery (*3*)

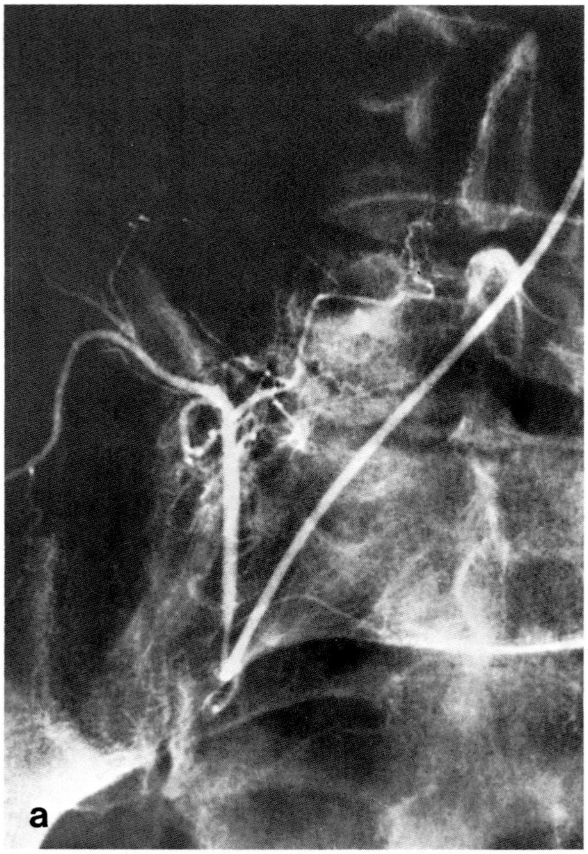

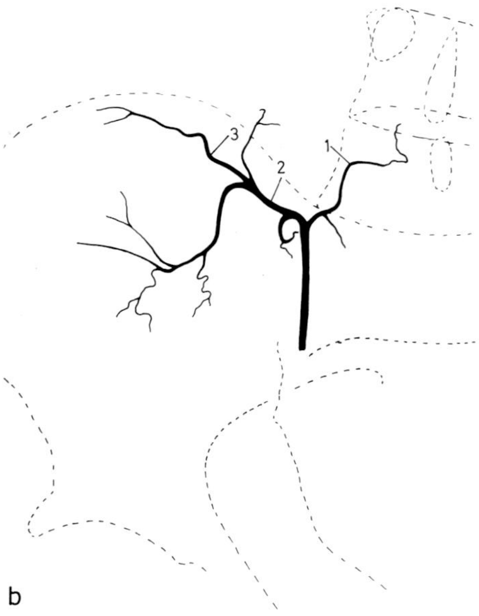

Fig. 11 a, b. Iliolumbar artery
1 lumbar branch
2 iliac branch
3 iliac crest artery

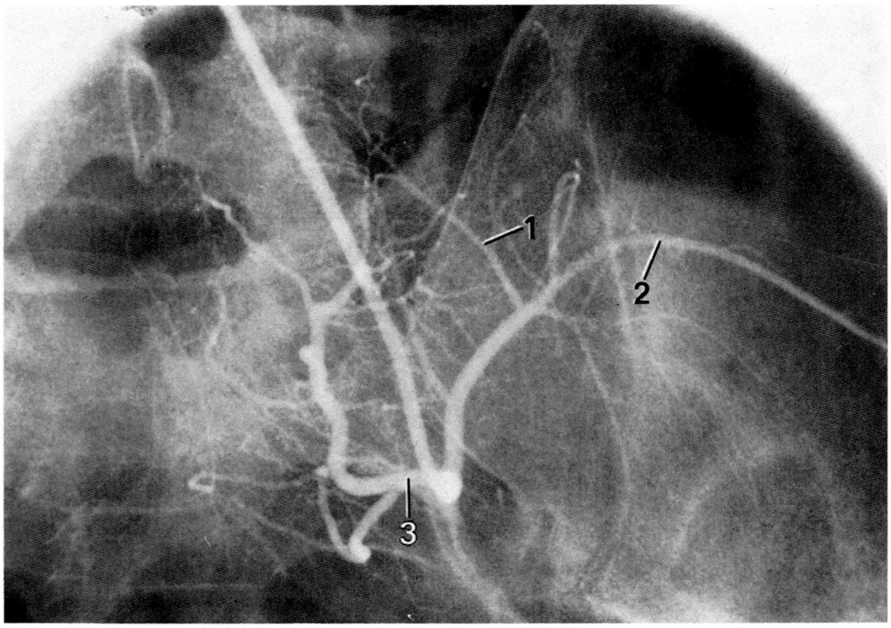

Fig. 12. Iliolumbar and sacral common trunk
1 lumbar branch
2 iliac branch
3 superior lateral sacral artery

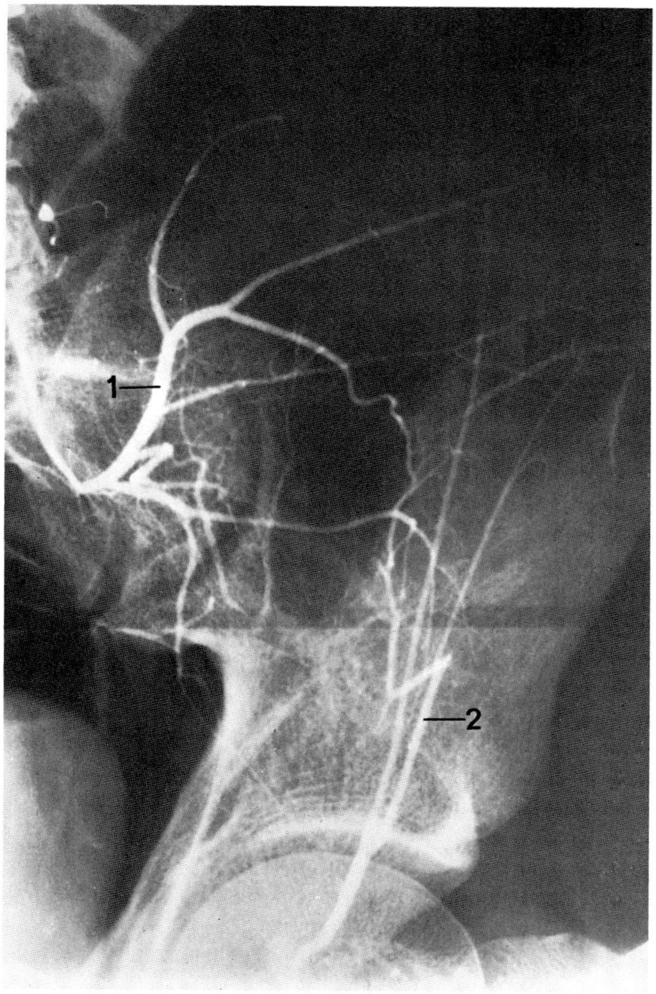

Fig. 13. Variation: isolated iliac branch (*1*) anastomosing with the deep iliac circumflex artery (*2*) branch of the external iliac artery on the anterior surface of the iliac muscle

---

The radiologic characteristics of the iliolumbar artery are:

a) It is the first branch of either posterior trunk or the hypogastric artery.
b) It runs upward facing the iliac wing, lateral to the hypogastric artery.
c) It divides into lateral and ascending branches at the level of L-5.

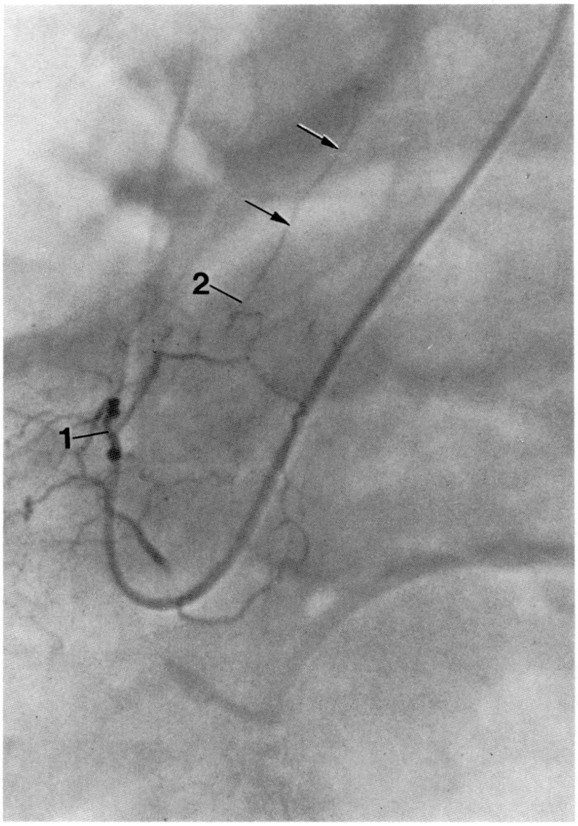

Fig. 14. A radicular artery (*2, arrow*) originating from an isolated lumbar artery (*1*)

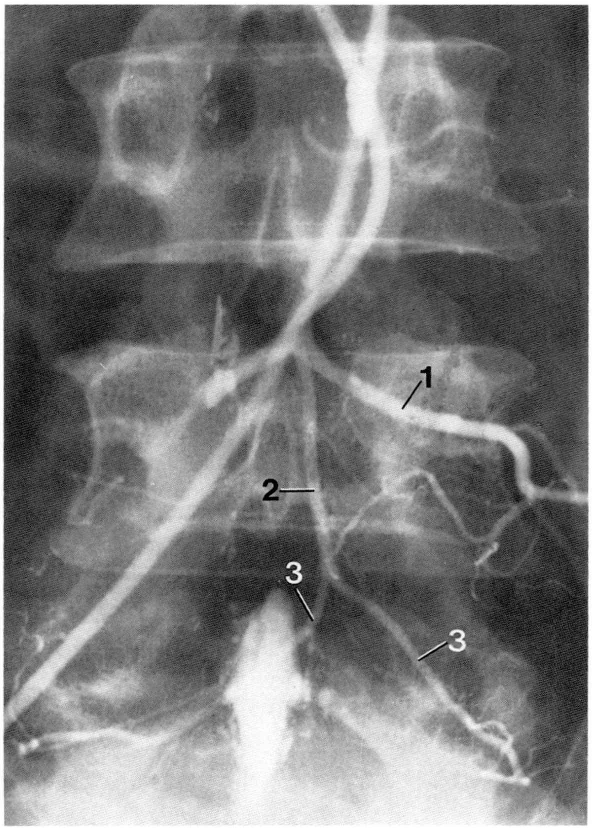

Fig. 15. Iliolumbar artery variation: absence of the lumbar branch. In that form the fifth lumbar artery (*3*) may arise from the aorta: In this case there is a common trunk between the left fourth lumbar artery (*1*) and the common vertical descending trunk for both fifth lumbar arteries (*3*) which divide in front of the L-5–S-1 intervertebral disc

Fig. 16 a–f. Main variations in origin of the lateral sacral arteries. **a** Separate origin of the inferior and superior lateral sacral arteries, arising from the posterior trunk (most frequent type). **b** Common trunk arising from the superior gluteal artery. **c** Separate origin of the superior and inferior sacral arteries arising from the common iliac artery. **d** Separate origin of these arteries arising from the anterior trunk. **e** Common trunk from the common iliac artery. **f** Superior sacral artery arising from the iliolumbar artery and inferior sacral artery arising from the superior gluteal artery ▷

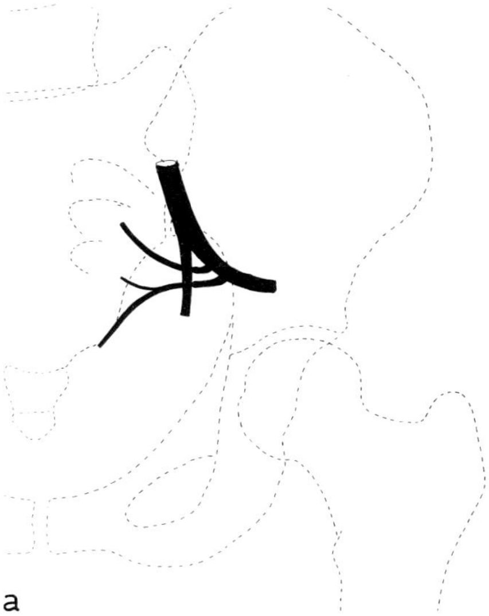

a

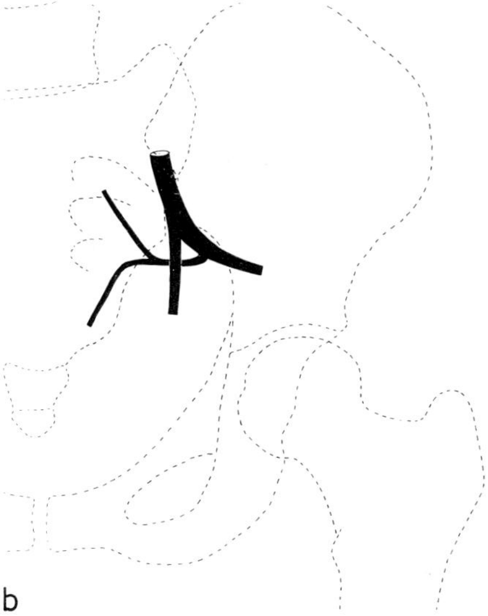

b

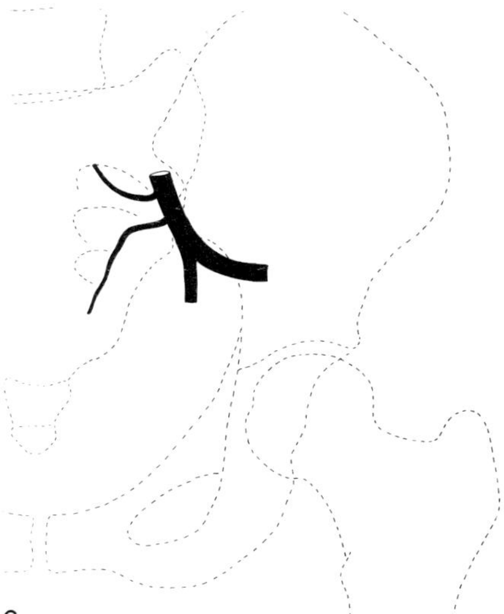

c

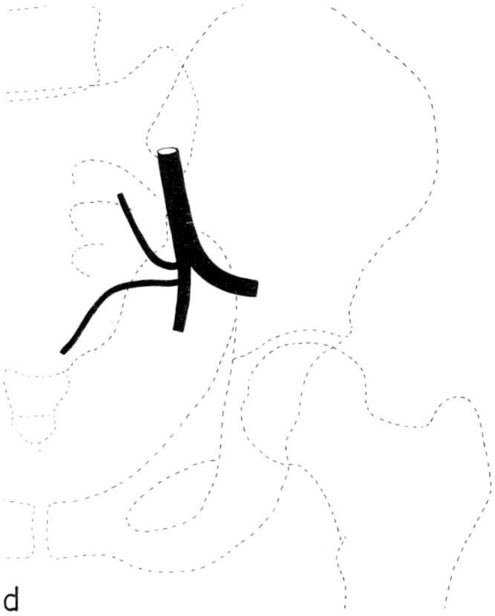

d

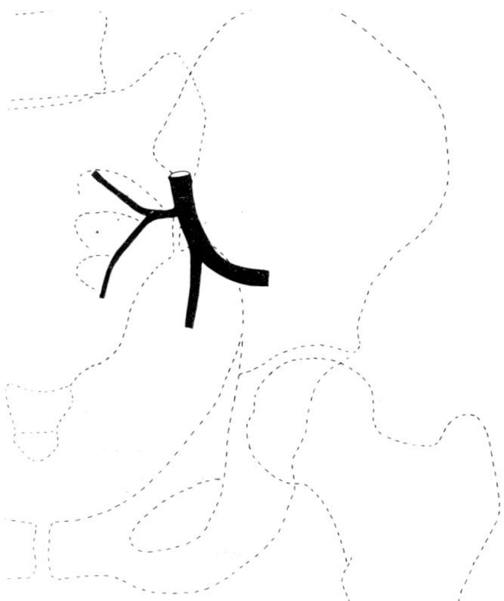

e

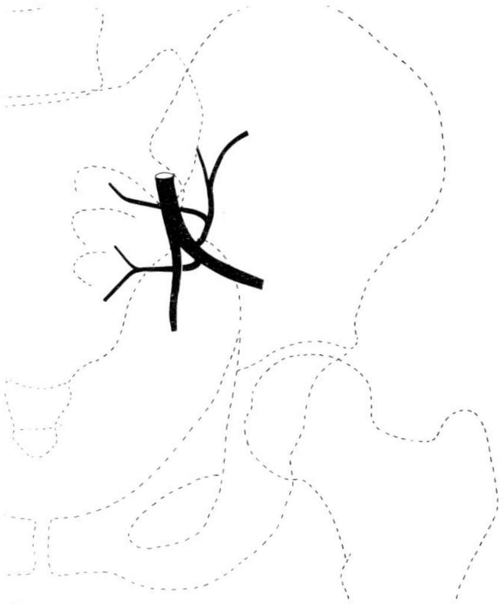

f

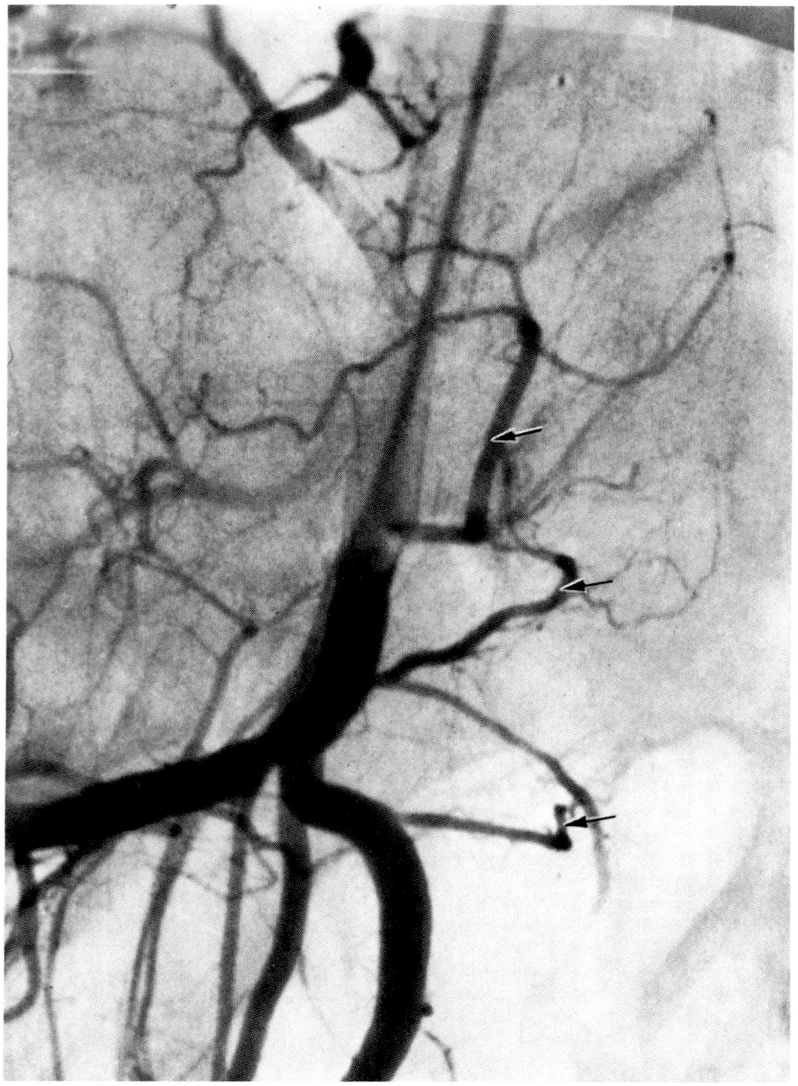

Fig. 17. Variation in the sacral lateral arteries: three separate arteries arising from the internal iliac, superior gluteal, and inferior gluteal arteries

The radiologic characteristics of the superior lateral sacral artery are that it takes a medial course toward the first anterior sacral foramen, in front of which it bends at a right angle and continues upward.

The radiologic characteristics of the inferior lateral sacral artery are:
An initial lateral course followed by bifurcation in front of the second anterior sacral foramen, giving an ascending branch and a descending branch which extends to the tip of the coccyx; and usually bilateral injection via anastomoses.

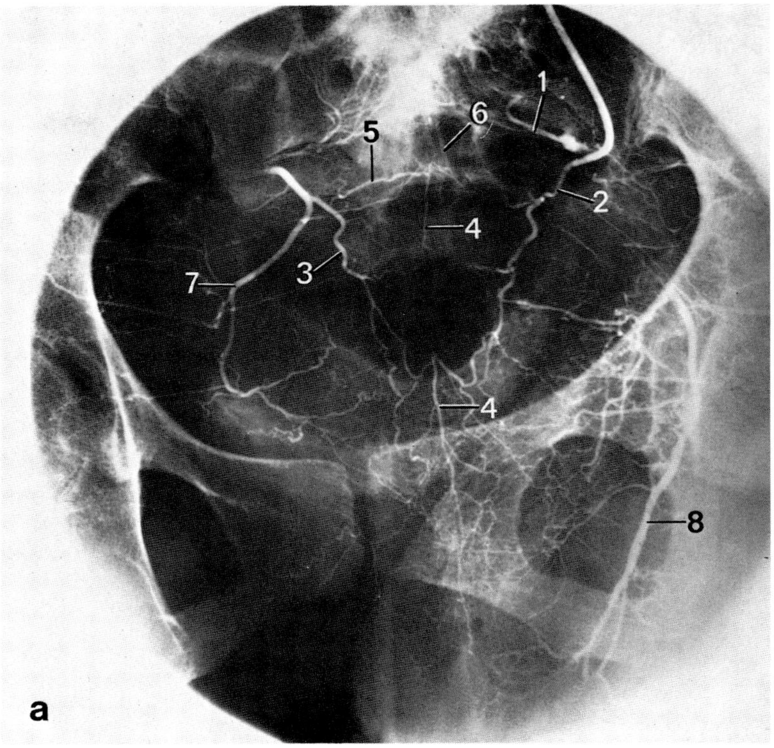

1 superior lateral sacral artery
2 inferior lateral sacral artery
3 contralateral inferior sacral artery
4 middle sacral artery
5 transverse presacral anastomoses
6 radicular branch
7 muscular branches usually arising from the inferior gluteal artery
8 internal pudendal artery

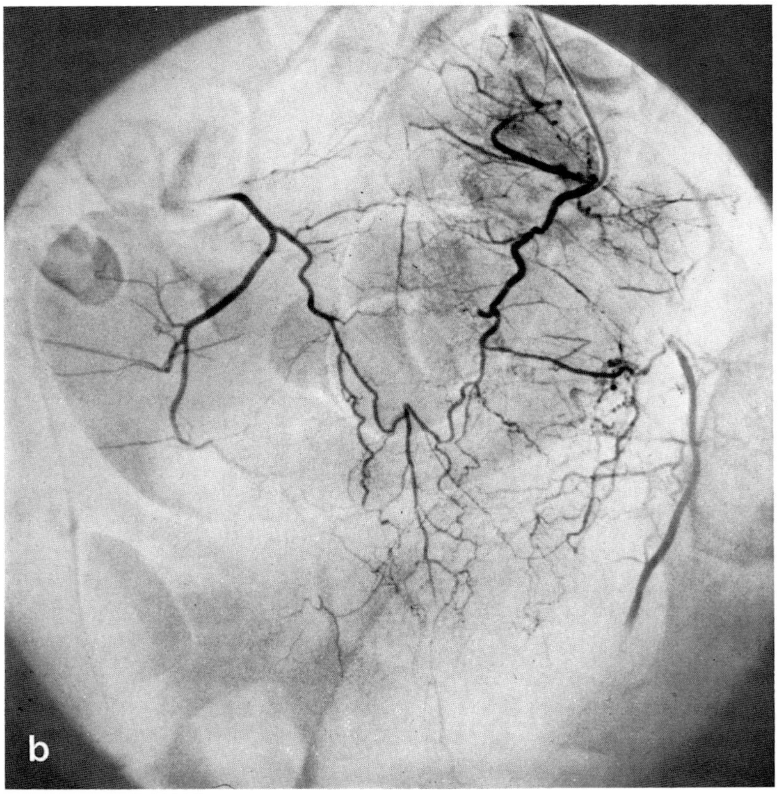

Fig. 18 a, b. Common trunk and anastomoses of the lateral sacral arteries

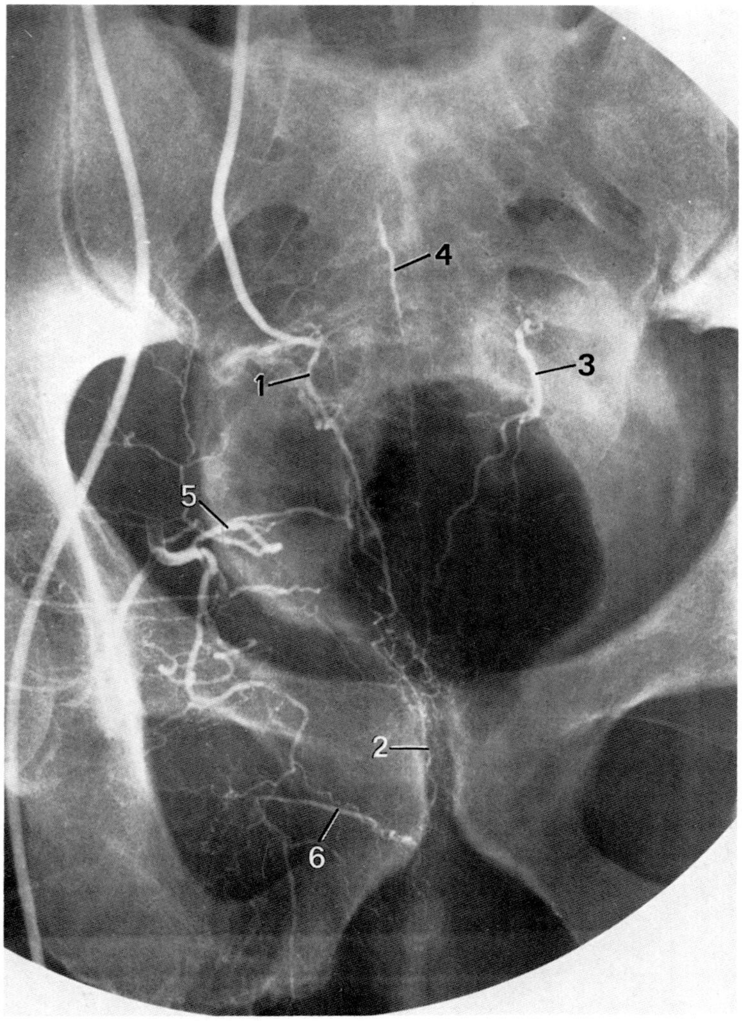

Fig. 19. Inferior lateral sacral artery and its anastomoses

1 inferior lateral sacral artery
2 inferior rectal (hemorrhoidal) artery
3 contralateral inferior lateral sacral artery
4 middle sacral artery
5 anastomotic branch to the inferior gluteal artery
6 internal pudendal artery

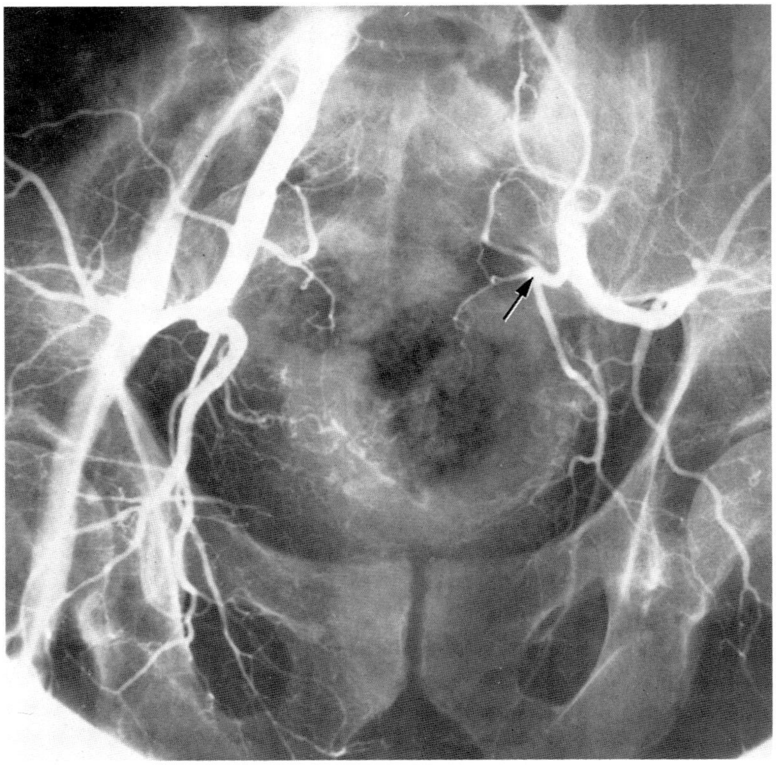

Fig. 20. Lateral sacral branches arising from the internal iliac artery. On the left side is a common trunk for the inferior gluteal and sacral arteries (*arrow*). A double inferior gluteal artery is present

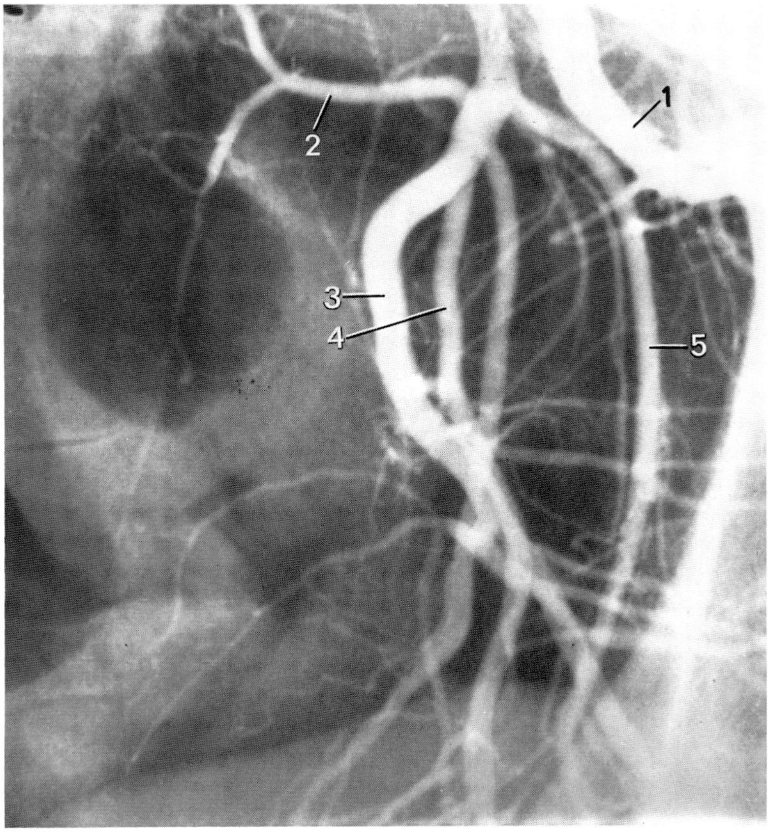

Fig. 21. Lateral sacral arteries arising from the anterior trunk
1 superior gluteal artery
2 lateral sacral artery
3 inferior gluteal artery
4 internal pudendal artery
5 obturator artery

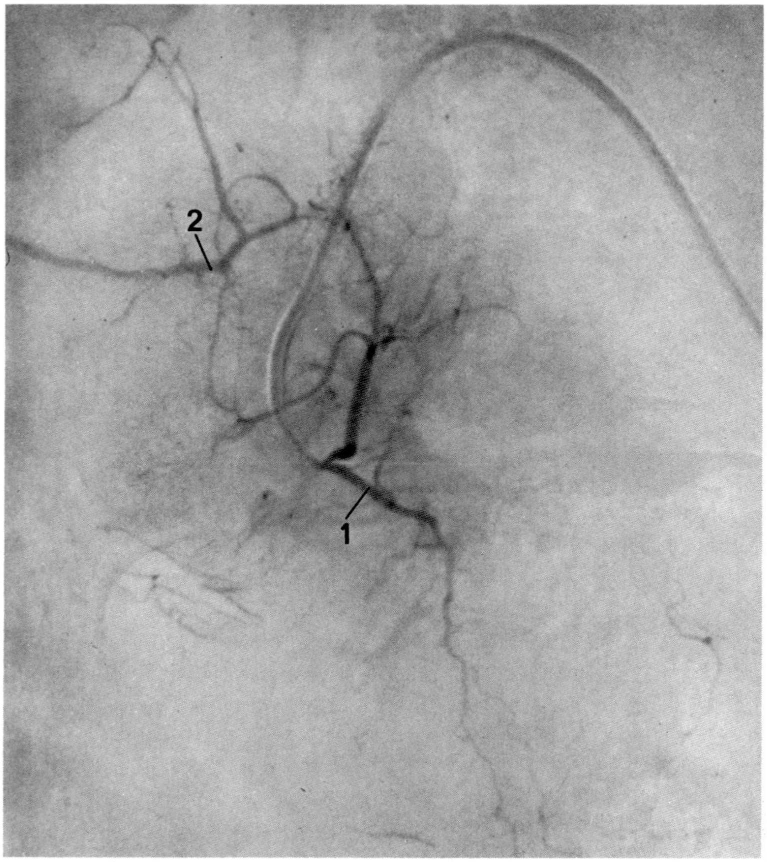

Fig. 22. Anastomoses of the lateral sacral (*1*) and the iliolumbar arteries (*2*)

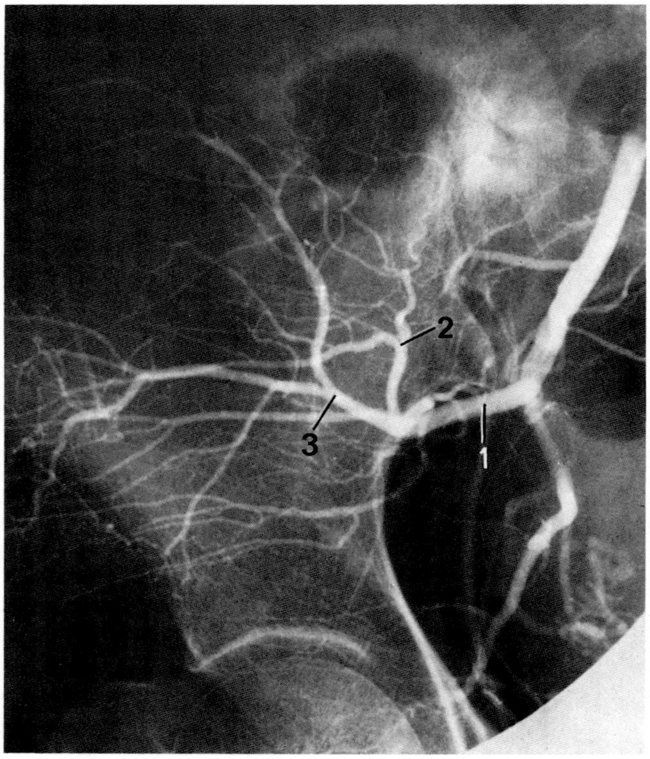

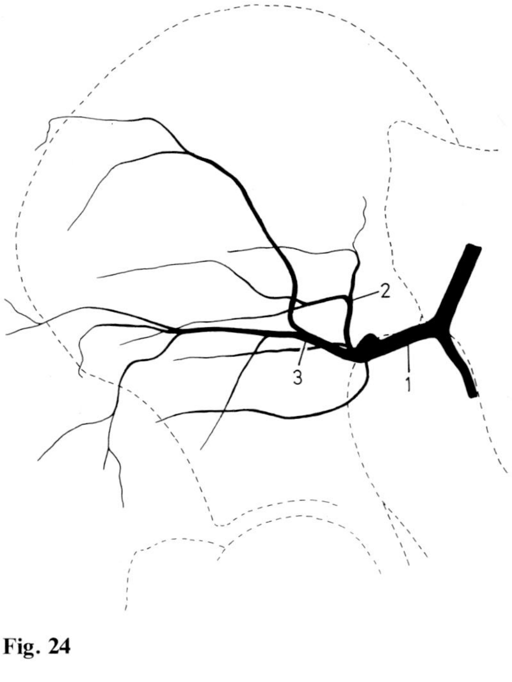

Fig. 24

◁ **Fig. 23**

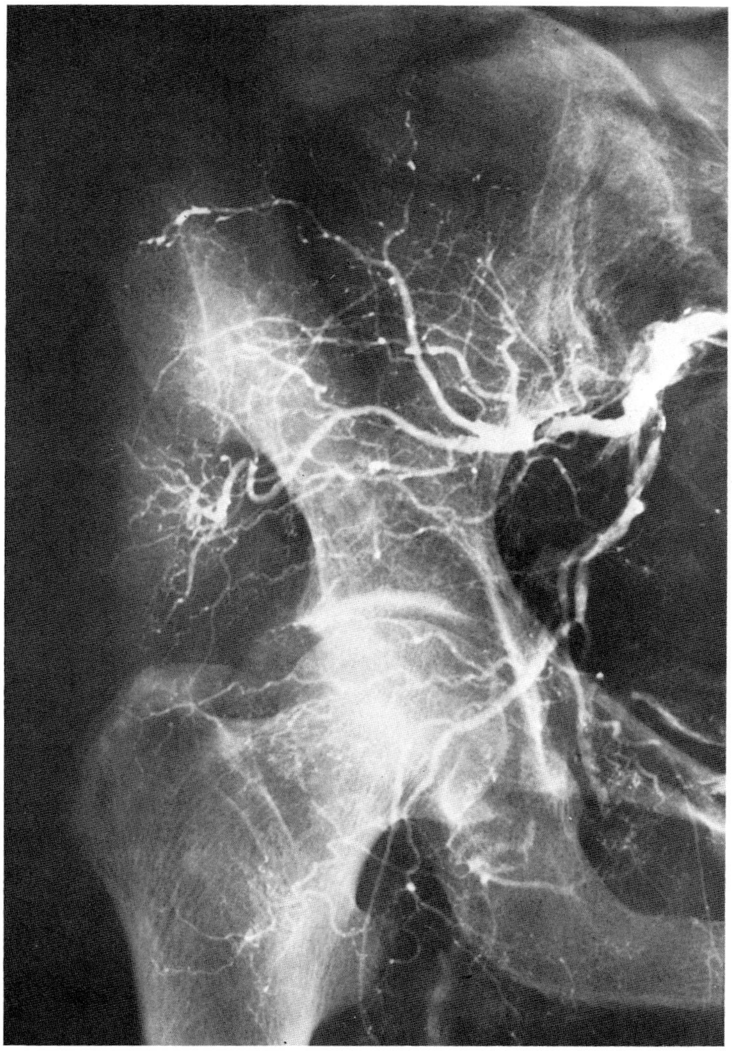

Fig. 25. Film of anatomic specimen

◁ **Fig. 23.** Superior gluteal artery
1 trunk of the artery
2 superficial branch
3 deep branch

◁ **Fig. 24.** Diagram of Fig. 23
1 trunk of the artery
2 superficial branch
3 deep branch

The radiologic characteristics of the superior gluteal artery are that it has a large caliber, an archlike shape, extends laterally, and ramifies into multiple branches opposite the iliac wing.

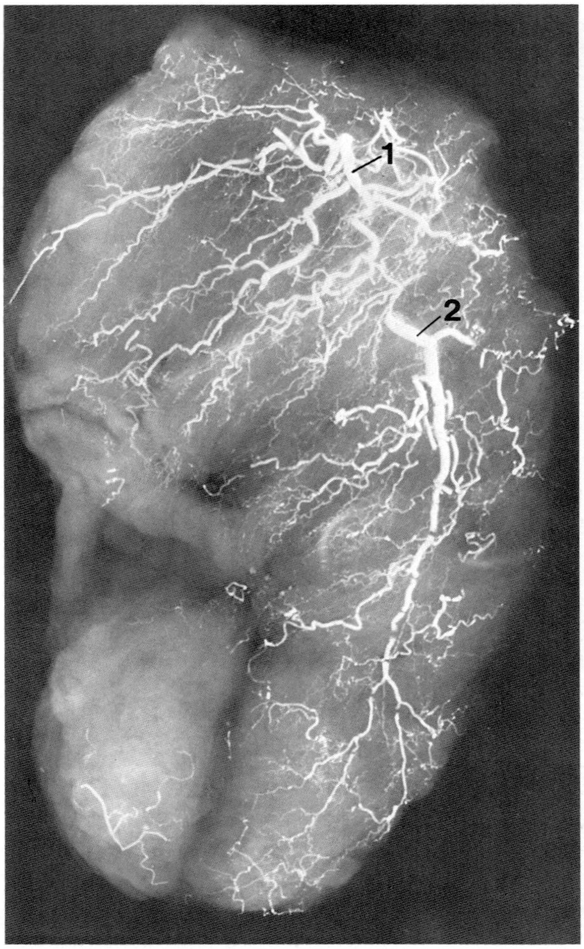

Fig. 26. Greatest gluteal muscle and its vessels
1 superficial branch of the superior gluteal artery
2 muscular branch arising from the inferior gluteal artery

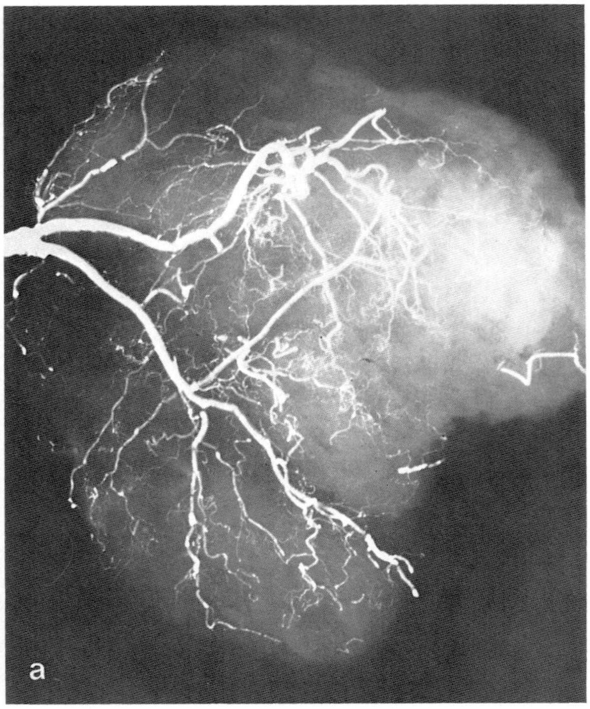

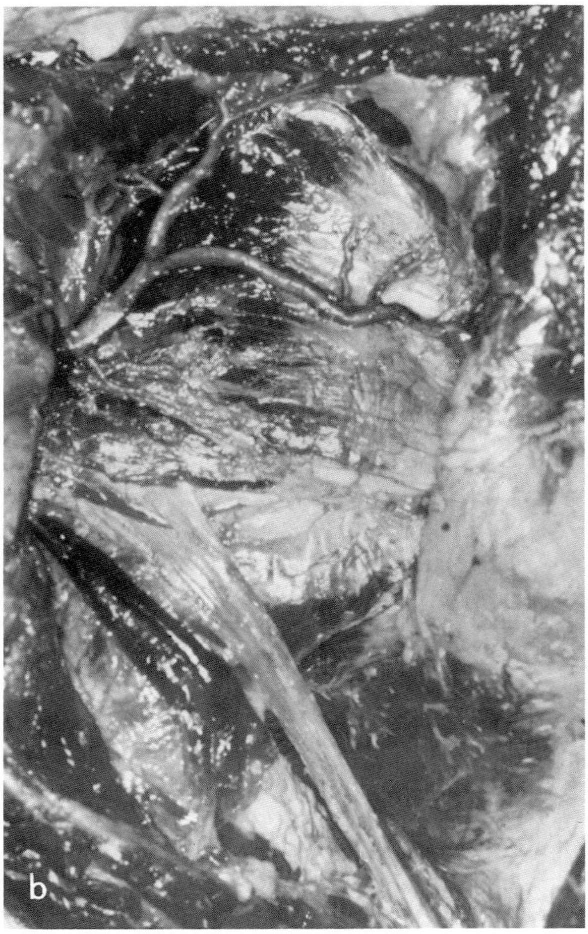

Fig. 27 a, b. Middle and least gluteal muscles with their vessels coming from the deep branch of the superior gluteal artery

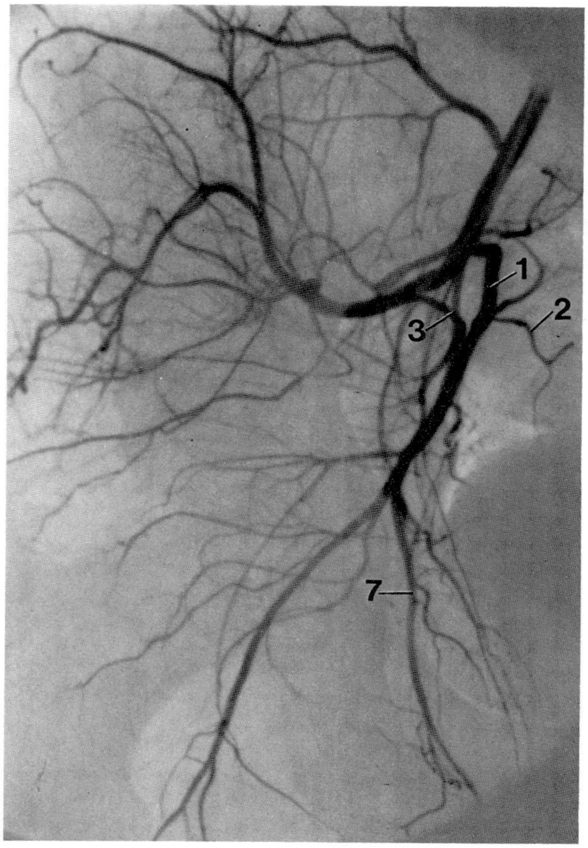

Fig. 28. Usual intrapelvic path taken by the inferior gluteal artery: it remains median to the other branches of the anterior trunk
1 inferior gluteal artery
2 lateral sacral artery
3 internal pudendal artery

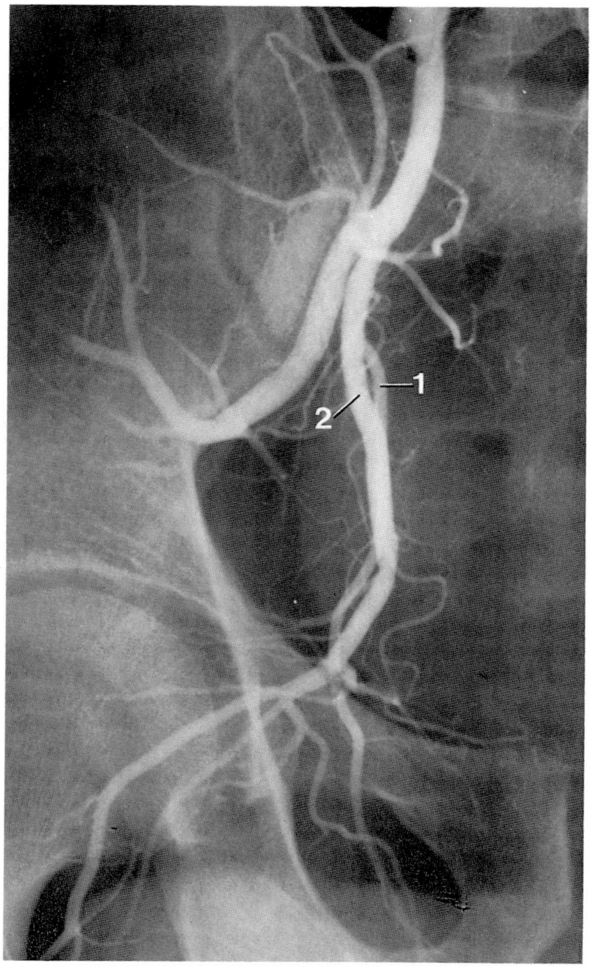

Fig. 29. Variations of the intrapelvic segment of the inferior gluteal artery (*2*) which is situated lateral to the internal pudendal artery (*1*)

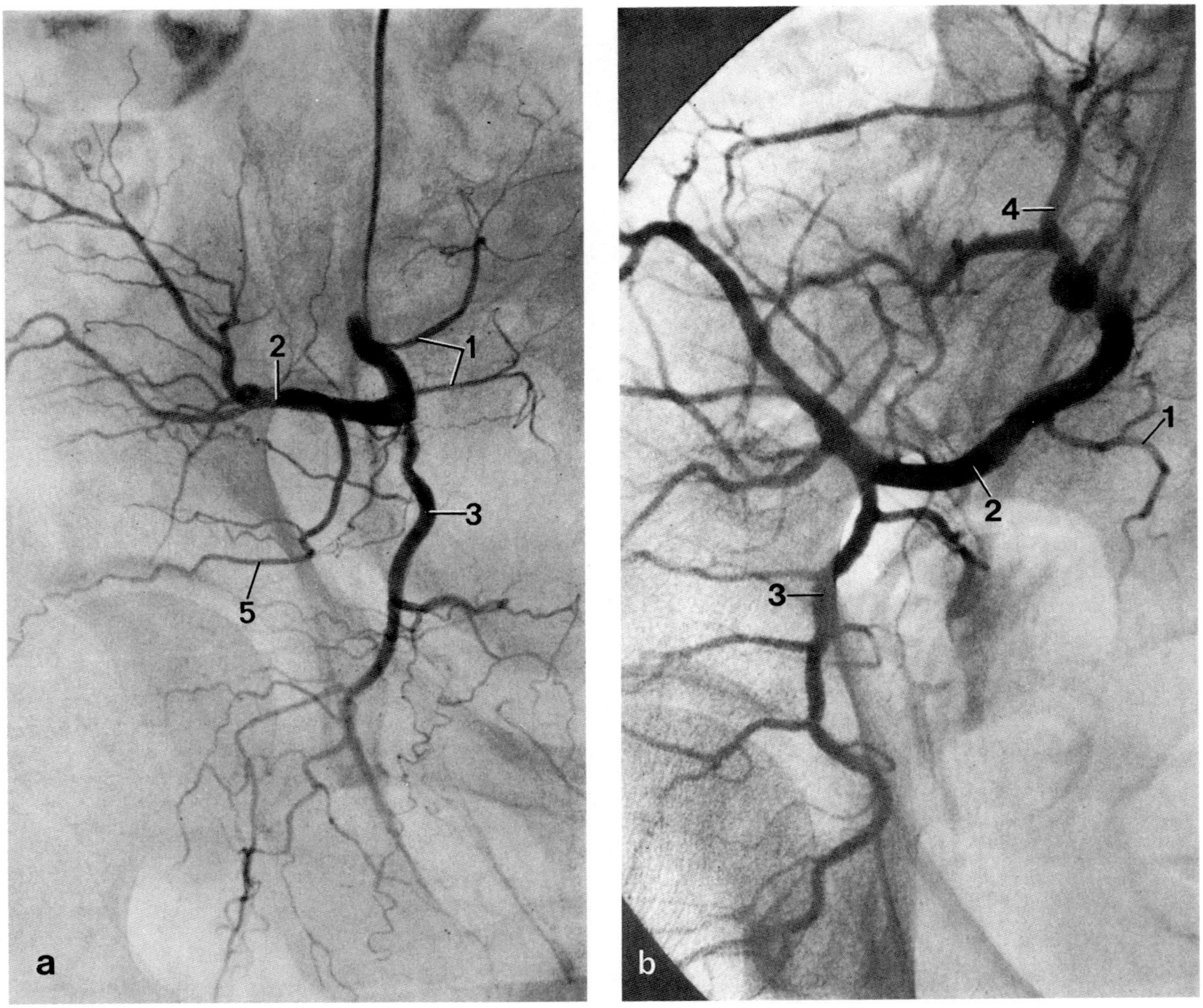

Fig. 30 a, b. Inferior gluteal artery arising from the posterior trunk
1 lateral sacral artery
2 superior gluteal artery
3 inferior gluteal artery
4 iliolumbar artery
5 inferior branch of the superior gluteal artery

The radiologic characteristics of the inferior gluteal artery are:
a) Variable intrapelvic course forming a semicircle which is open laterally.
b) Terminates behind the neck of the femur where it breaks up into a number of diverging branches that course in a downward lateral manner.

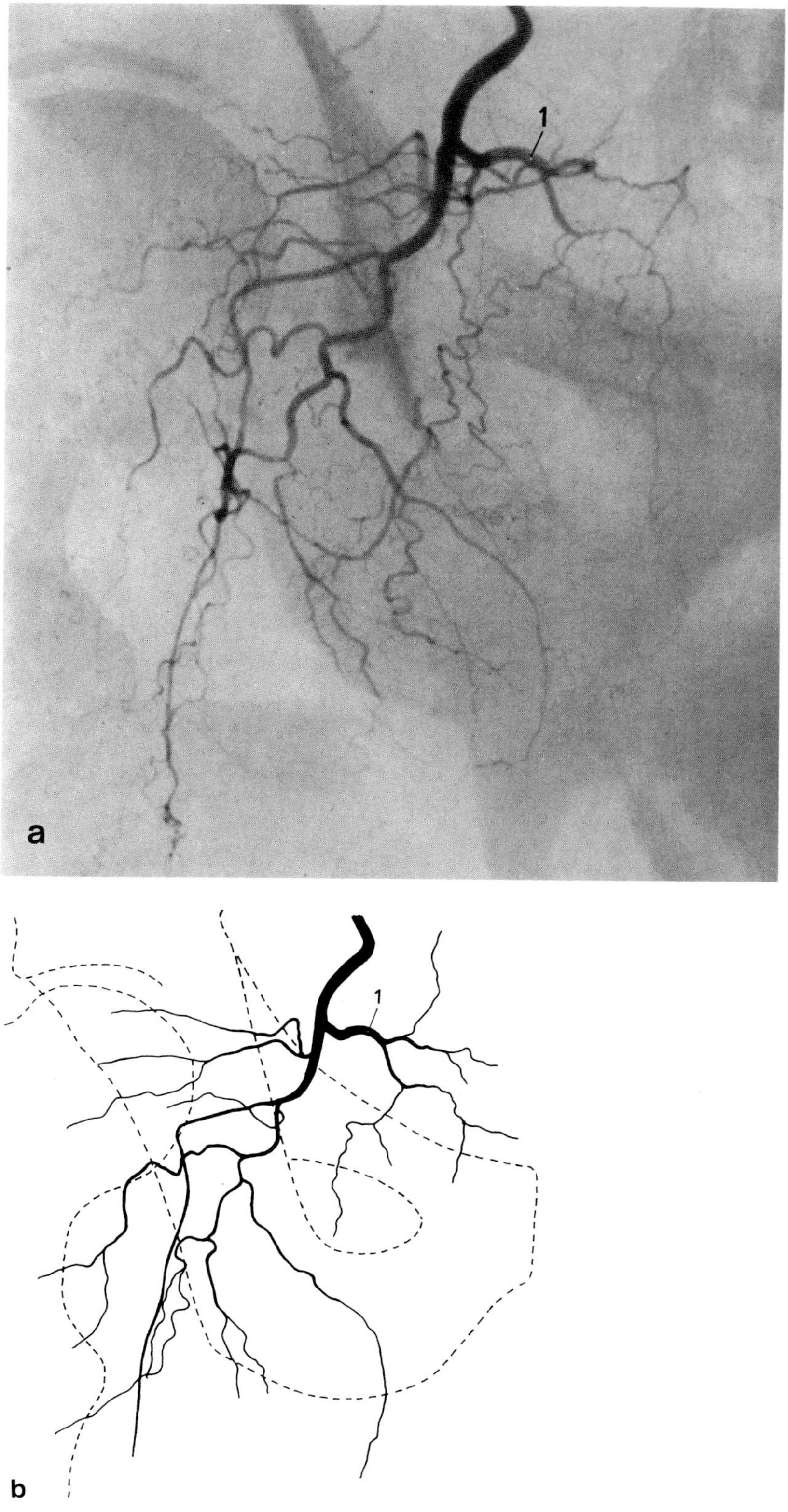

Fig. 31. Muscular branches from inferior gluteal artery, in particular an internal ramus for the piriform muscle (*1*)

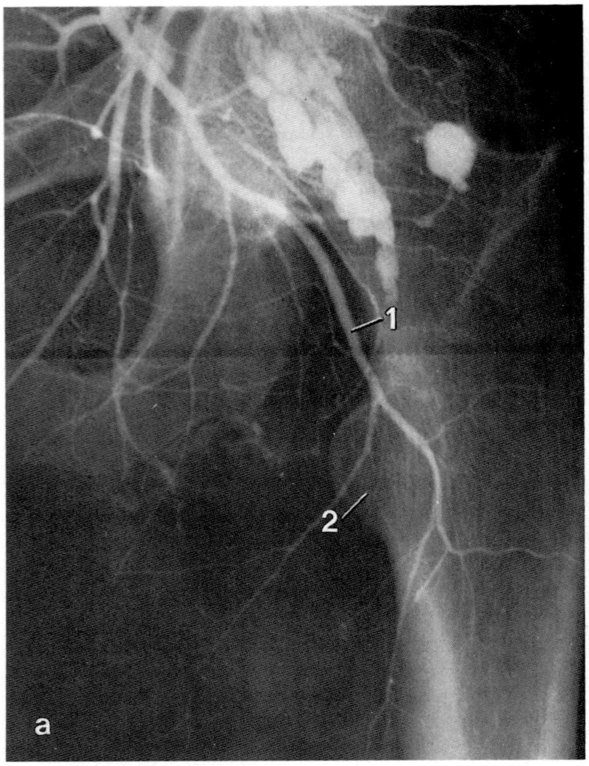

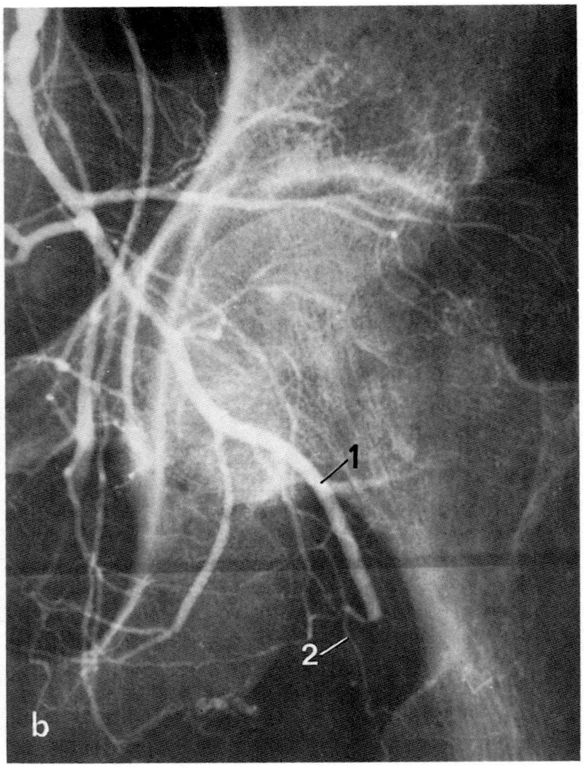

Fig. 32. The sciatic nerve artery is difficult to visualize in normal cases (**a**) but it may become visible following embolization of the main branches of the inferior gluteal artery (**b**)

1 descending branch of the inferior gluteal artery
2 sciatic nerve artery

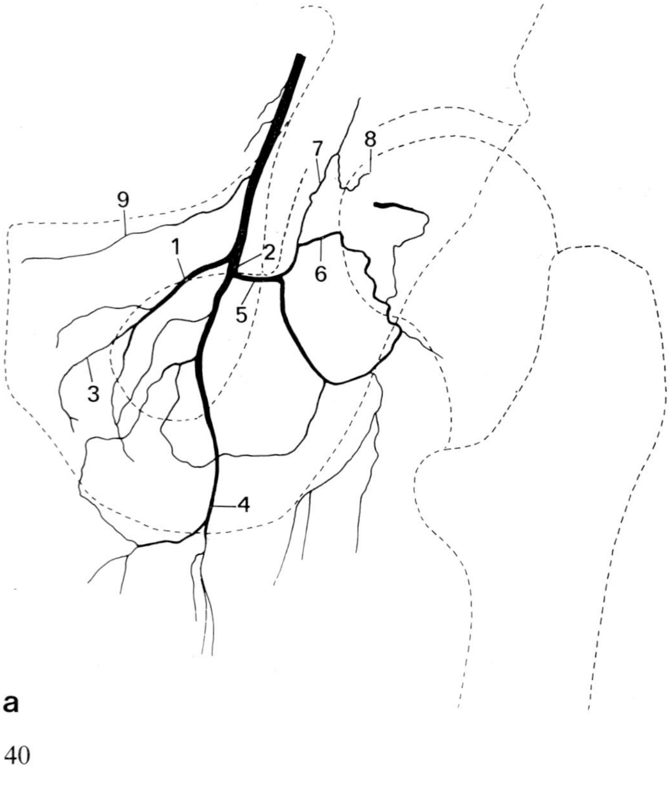

a

Fig. 33 a, b. Obturator artery and its branches
1 branch for the obturator muscle
2 posterior branch
3 cutaneous branch for the scrotum
4 branch for the medial part of the thigh
5 acetabular branch
6 articular branch
7 acetabular ramus
8 foveal ramus
9 retropubic ramus

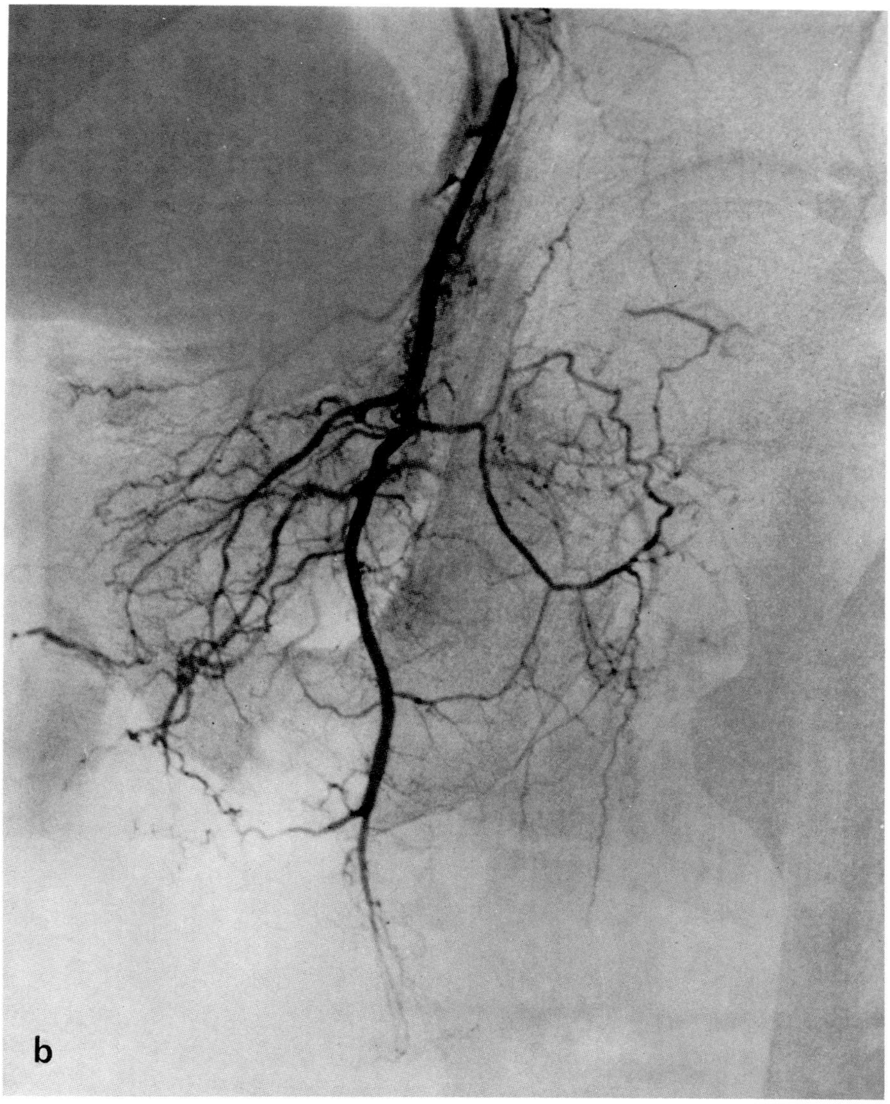

Fig. 33b

The radiologic characteristics of the obturator artery are that it courses along the brim of the pelvis, then bifurcates above the obturator notch into two branches which run along the course of the ischiopubic and iliopubic rami.

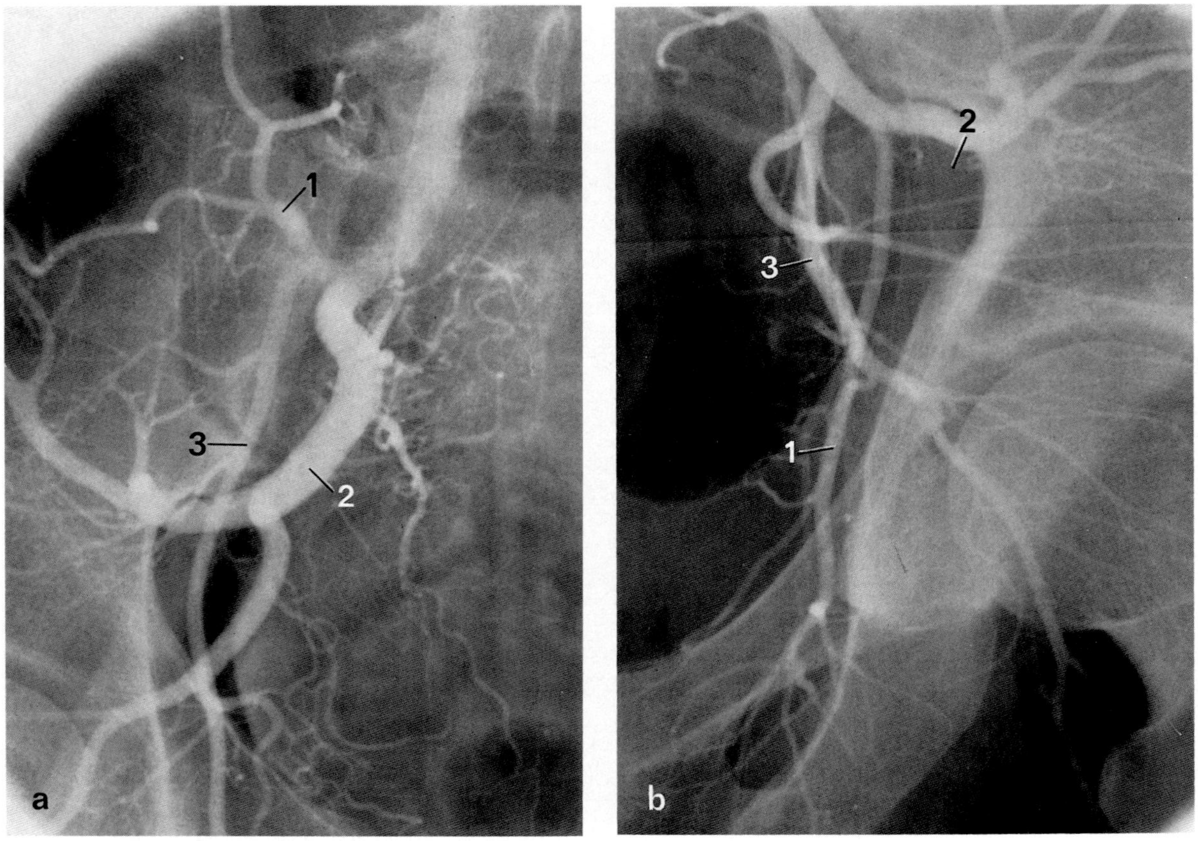

Fig. 34 a, b. Variations in the origin of the obturator artery. **a** From the iliolumbar artery (*1*), posterior trunk (*2*), obturator artery (*3*)
b From the posterior trunk:
1 obturator artery
2 superior gluteal artery
3 inferior gluteal artery

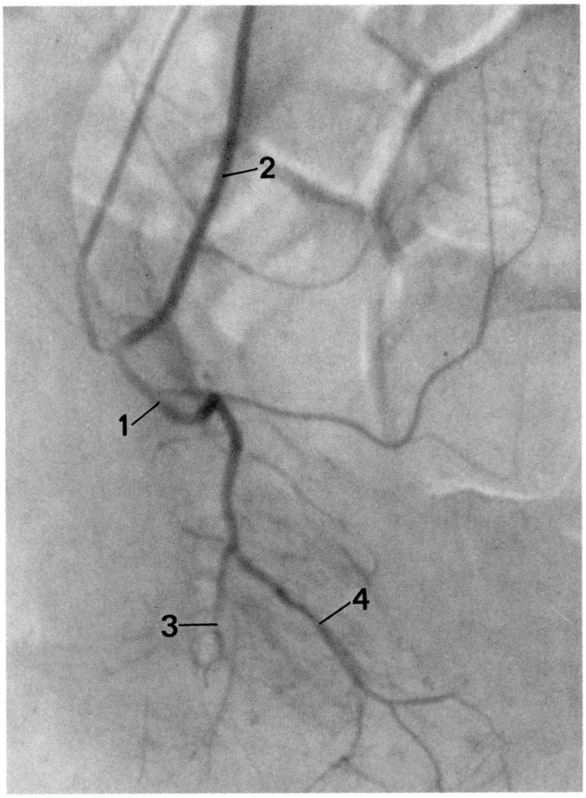

Fig. 35. Obturator artery (*1*) arising from the epigastric artery (*2*). It divides into two branches, external (*3*) and internal (*4*) above the obturator foramen

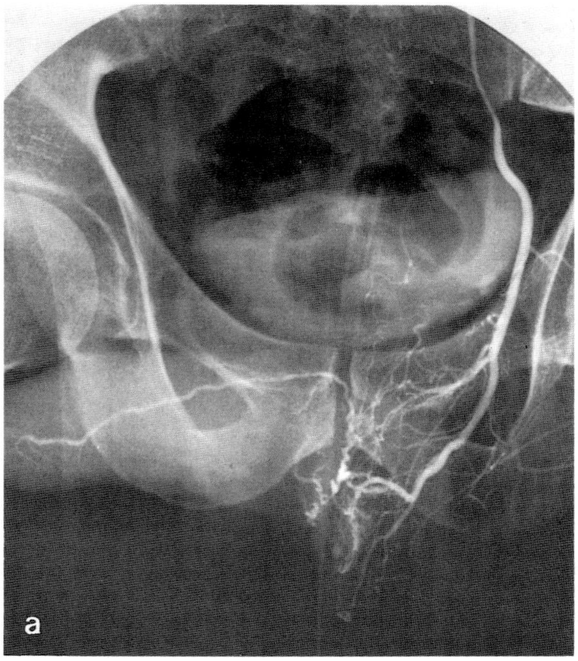

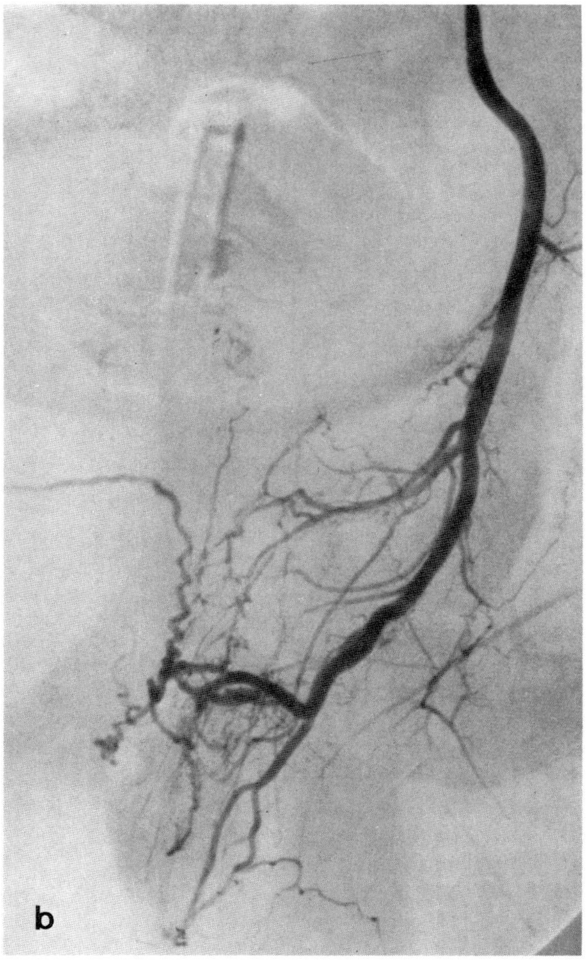

Fig. 36 a–c. Characteristic downward medial course of the internal pudendal artery ending on the midline, and giving a dense opacification of the bulb of penis
1 inferior rectal artery opacifying the arteries of the anal canal (*2*)
3 perineal artery
4 artery of the bulb giving the dorsal artery of the penis (*5*)
6 blood supply of the glans

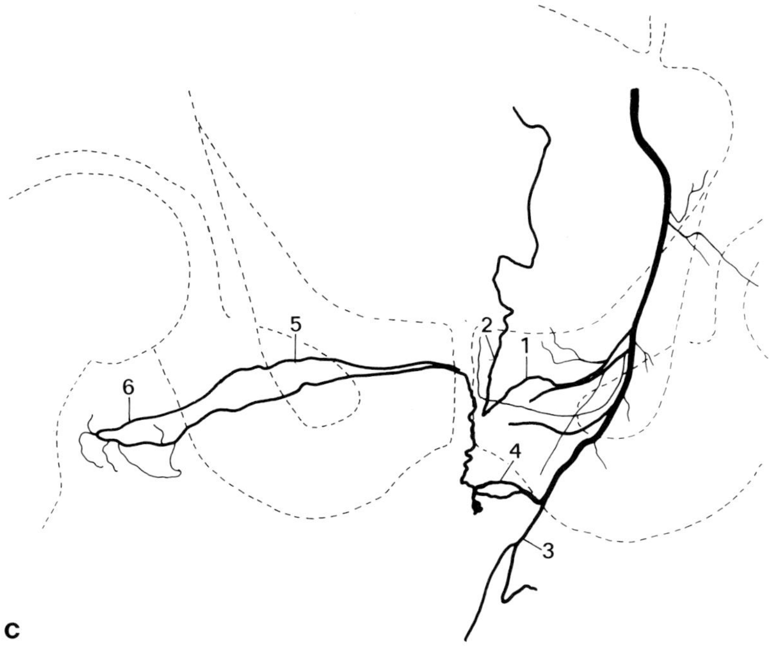

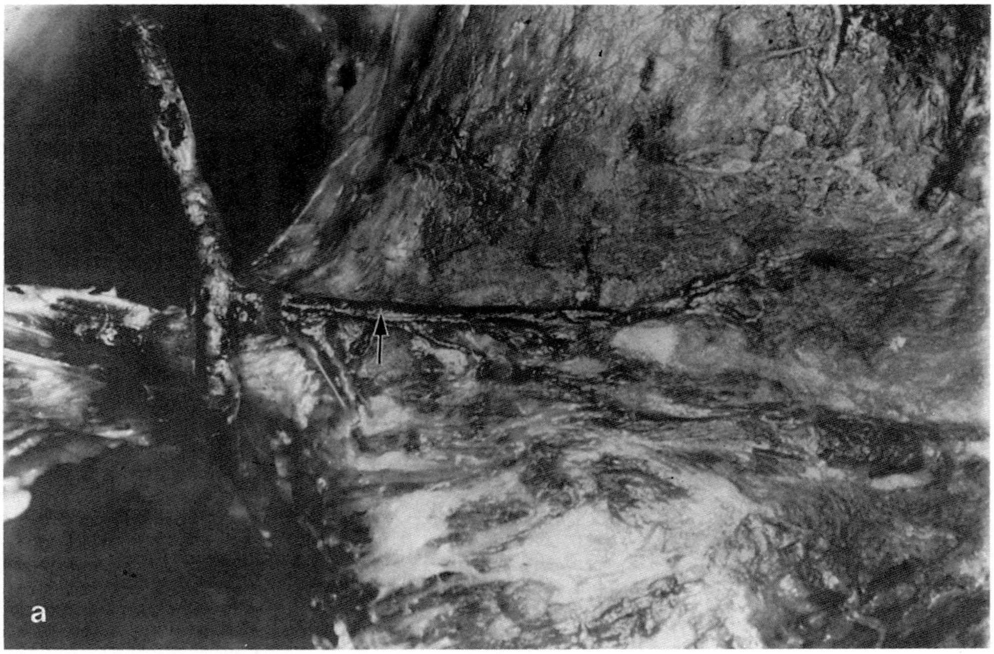

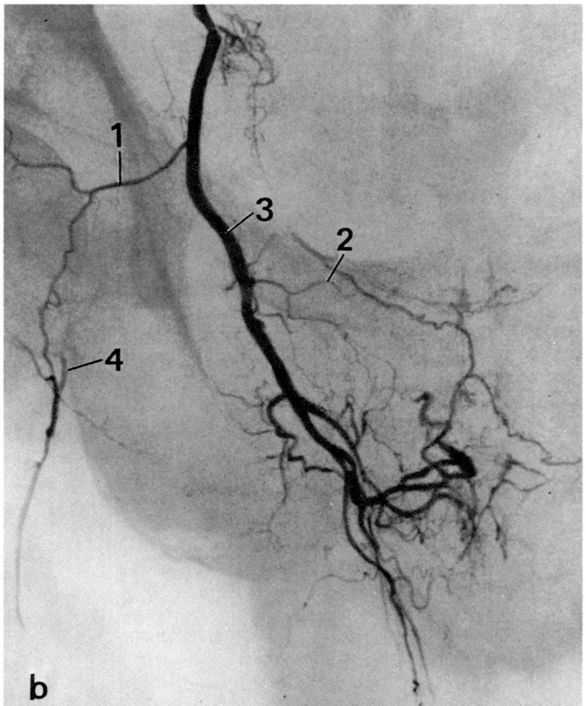

Fig. 37 a, b. Internal pudendal artery.
a Anatomic specimen, posterior view: ischial branch (*arrow*)
b Parietal branches
1 artery of the acetabulum and gemellus muscle
2 retropubic branch
3 ischial branch
4 anastomoses with inferior gluteal artery

The radiologic characteristics of the internal pudenal artery are:

a) A downward medial intrapelvic course.
b) It becomes horizontal just below the symphysis and it terminates on the midline.
c) Dense opacification at the base of the corpus bulbocavernosum.

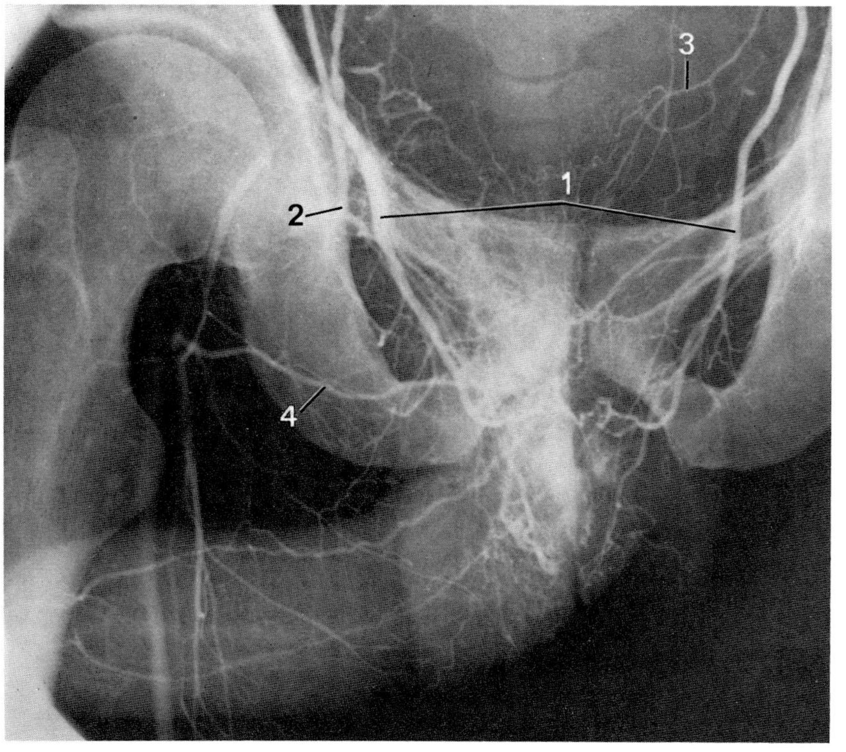

Fig. 38. Arterial anastomoses with other branches of the hypogastric artery
1 internal pudendal artery
2 obturator artery
3 middle rectal artery
4 external pudendal artery

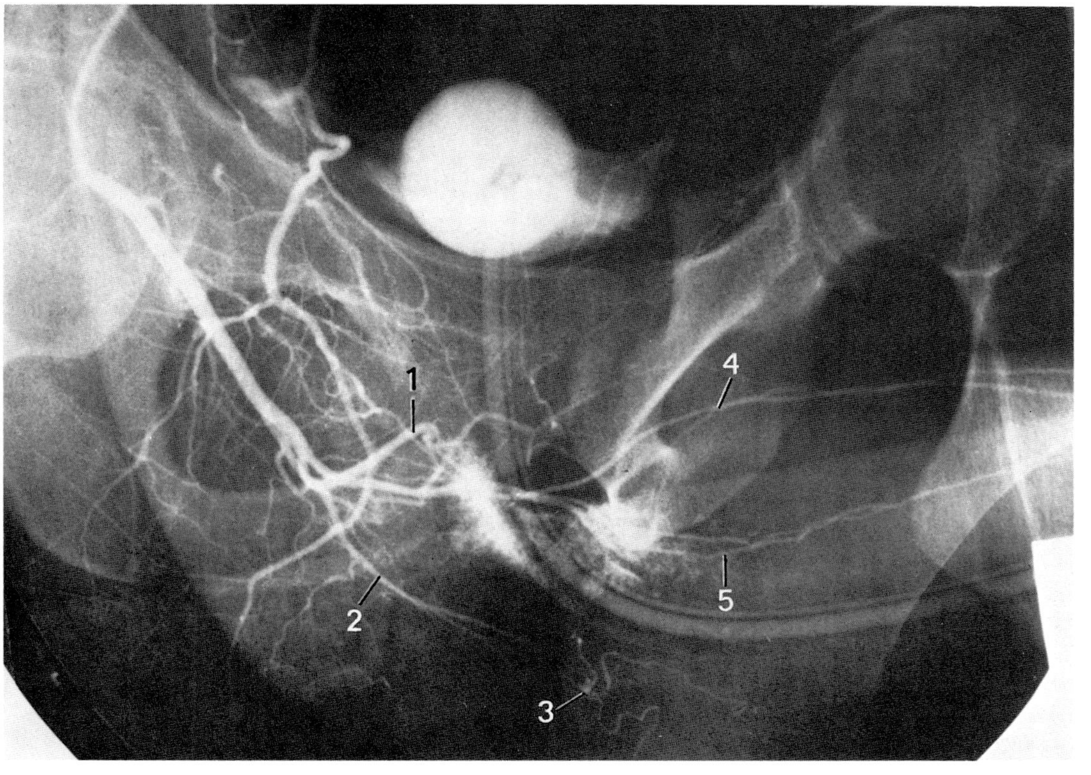

Fig. 39. Artery of the bulb (*1*) with retrograde injection of perineal artery (*2*). Vascularization of scrotum (*3*). Homo- and contralateral artery of penis (*4, 5*)

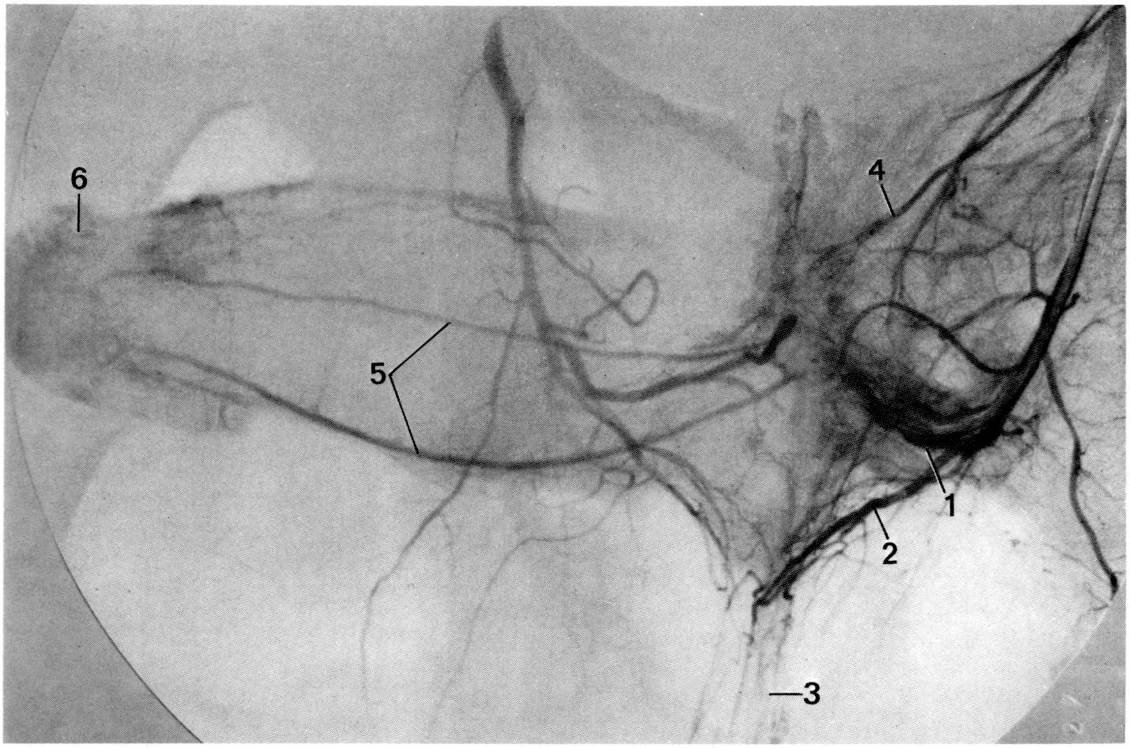

Fig. 40. Internal pudendal artery in male
1 bulbar artery
2 perineal artery
3 scrotal artery
4 branches for anal canal
5 artery of penis
6 opacification of glans peni

▽ **Fig. 41.** Venous drainage in the male
1 corpus cavernosum
2 corpus spongiosum
3 corpus bulbocavernosum

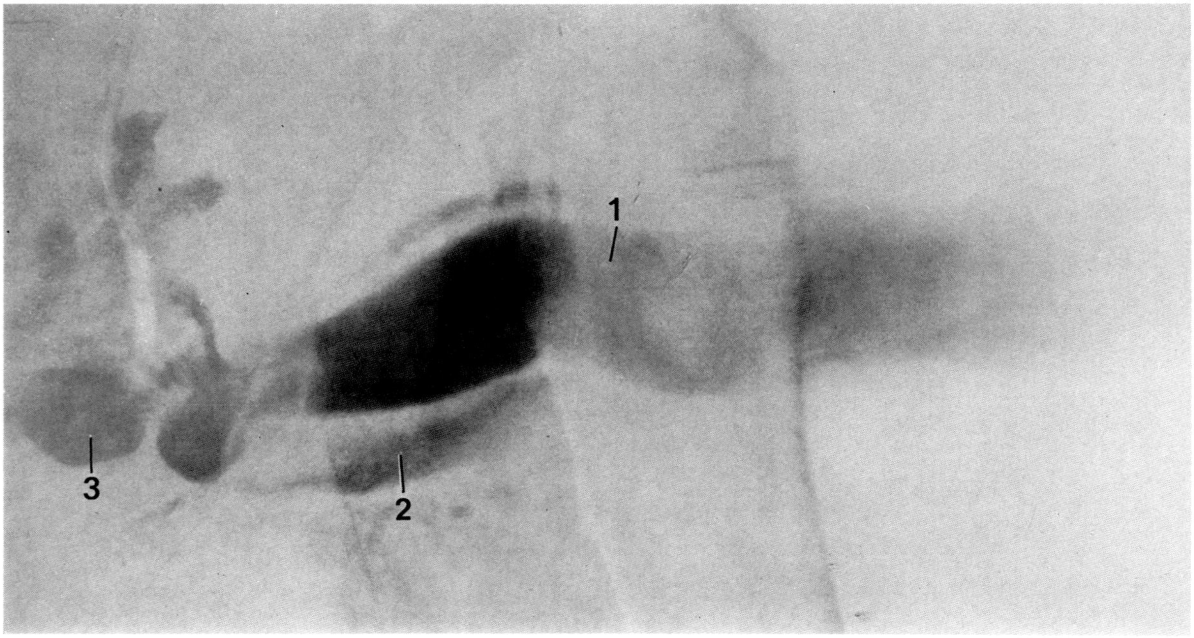

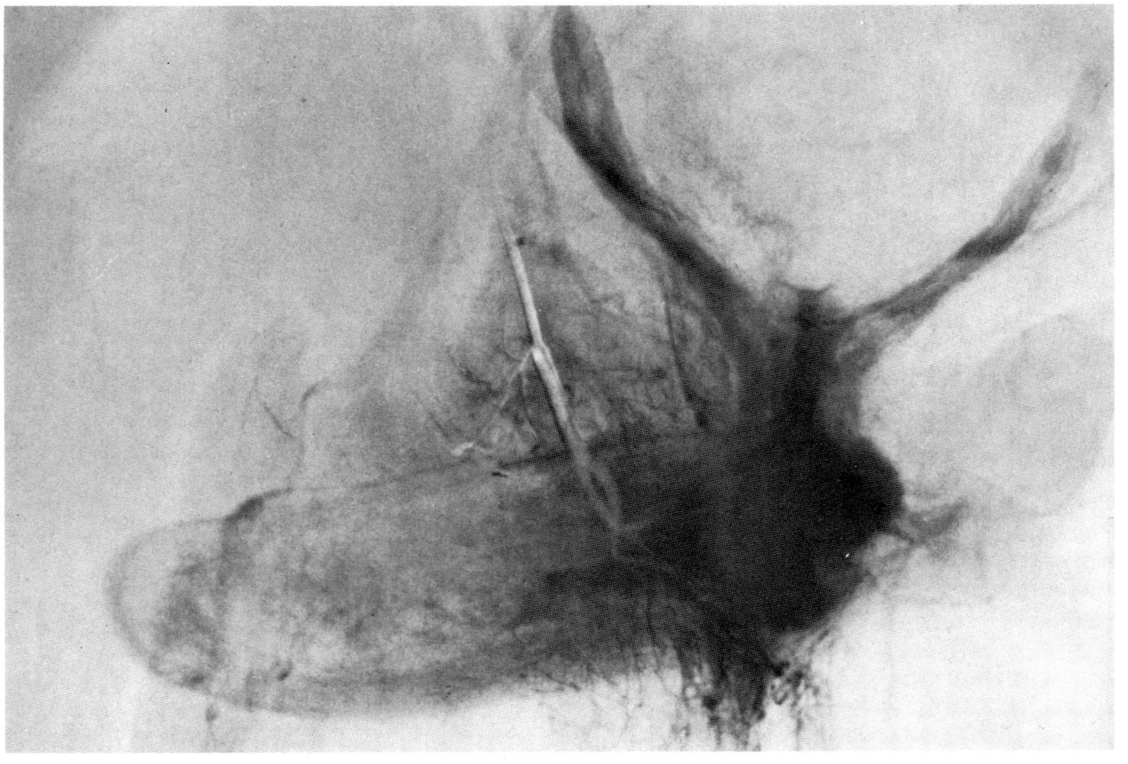

Fig. 42. Venous drainage into the prevesical and laterovesical plexi

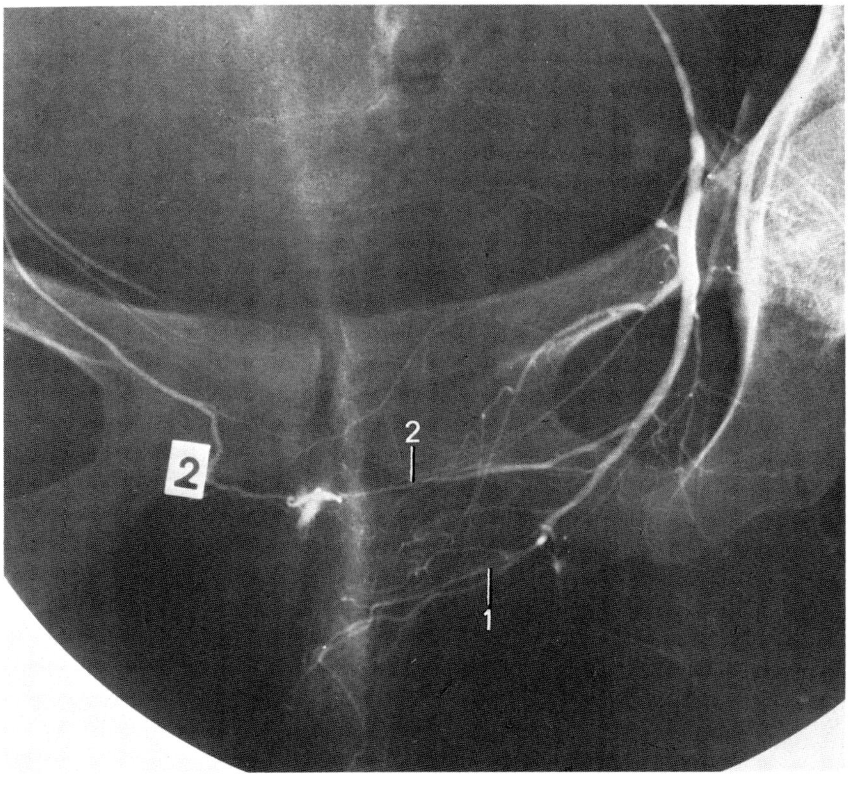

Fig. 43. Internal pudendal artery in the female
1 perineal artery
2 posterior labial branches

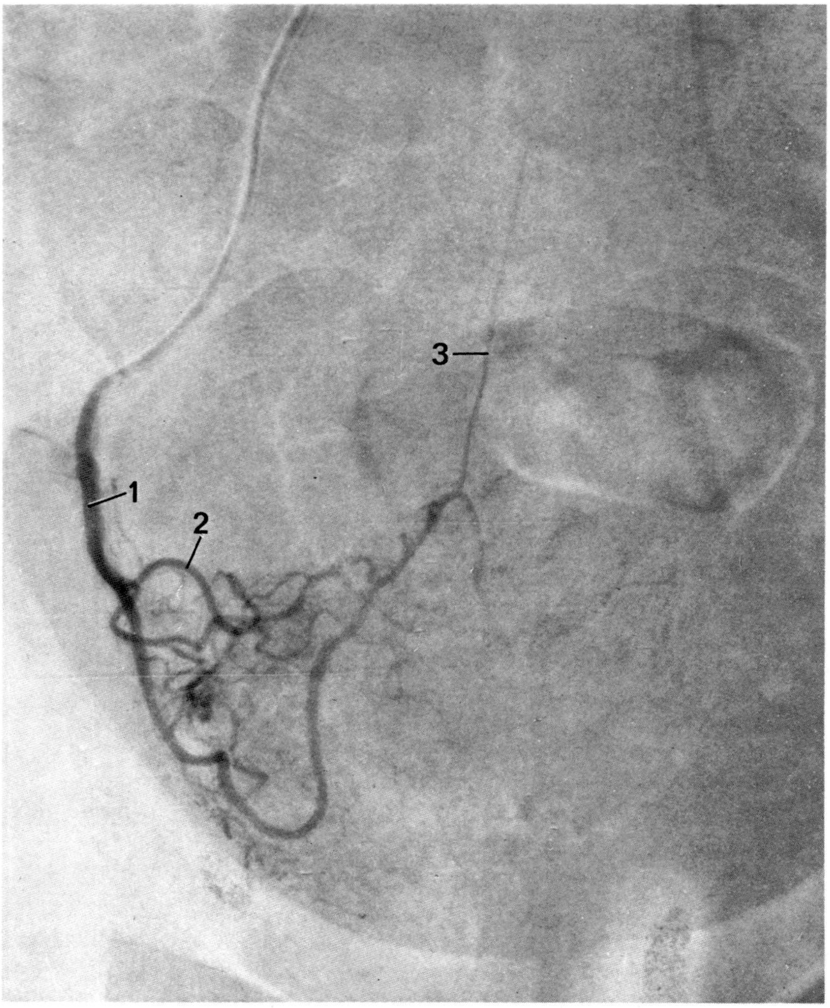

Fig. 44. Umbilical artery
1 trunk
2 superior vesical artery
3 umbilical segment

The radiologic characteristics of the umbilical artery are:

a) Empty bladder: suprapubic, downward, medial course.
b) Full bladder: course typically downward and median, then takes a sharp turn. Terminates by numerous inferiorly concave branches. The superior vesical branches course along the top of the bladder.

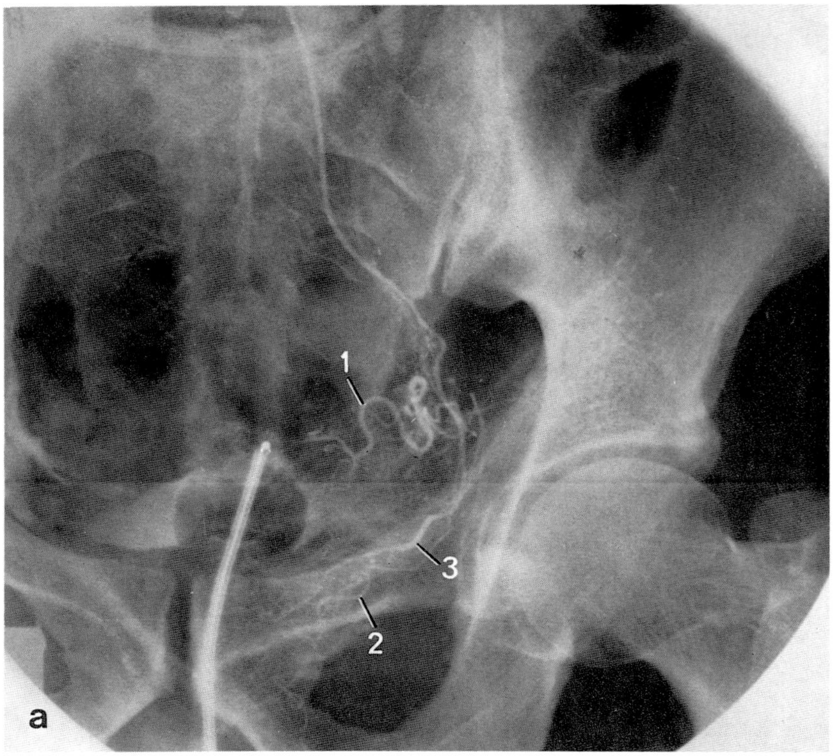

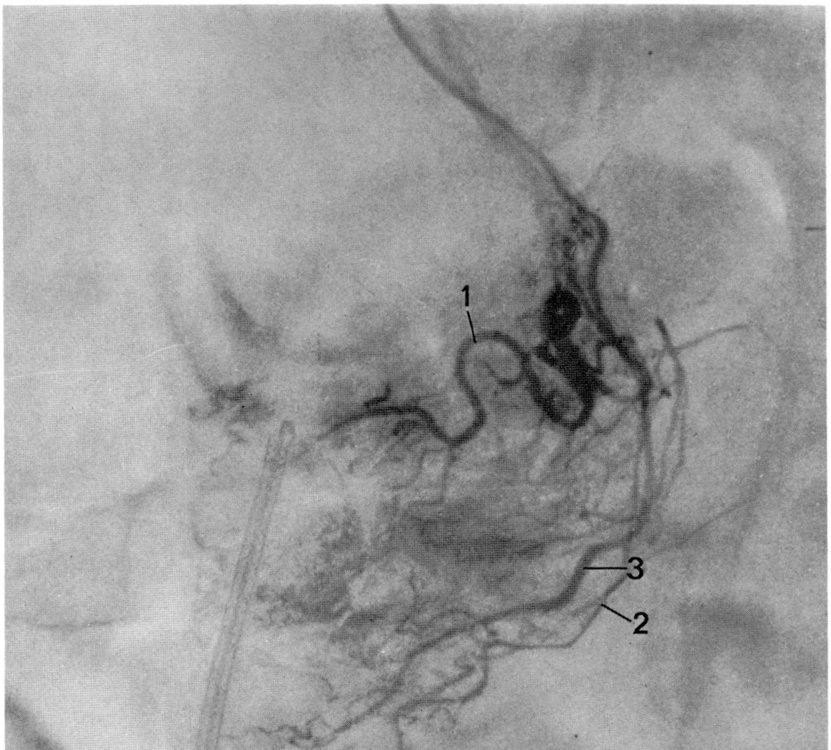

Fig. 45 a, b. Inferior vesical and prostatic arteries
1 inferior vesical artery
2 deferential artery
3 prostatic artery

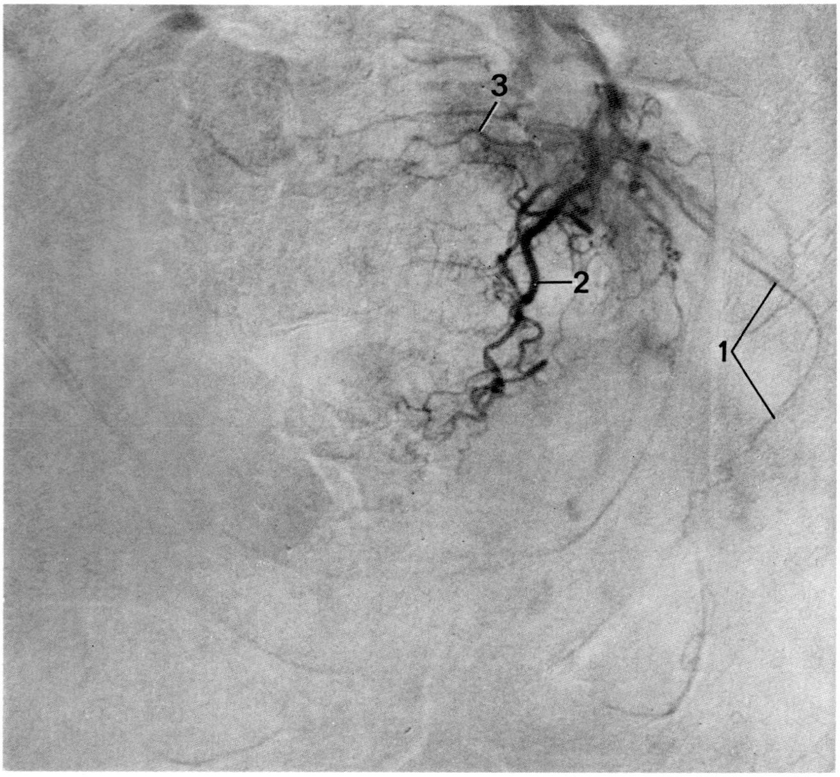

Fig. 46. Genitovesical artery
1 deferential artery
2 seminal vesicle branch
3 lateral vesical artery

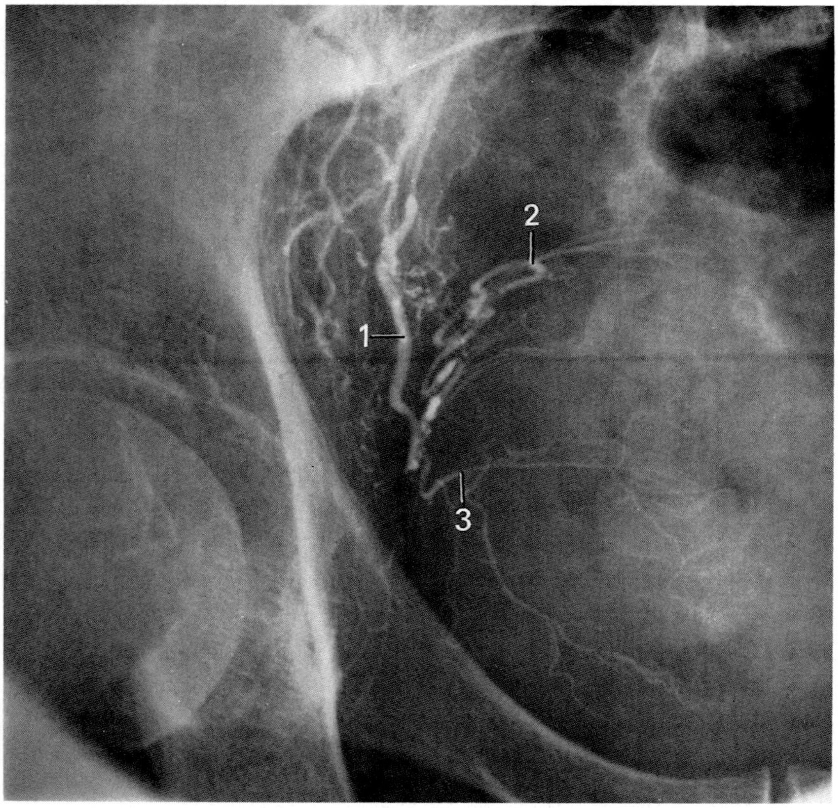

Fig. 47. Umbilical artery
1 arterial trunk
2 superior vesical artery
3 lateral vesical artery

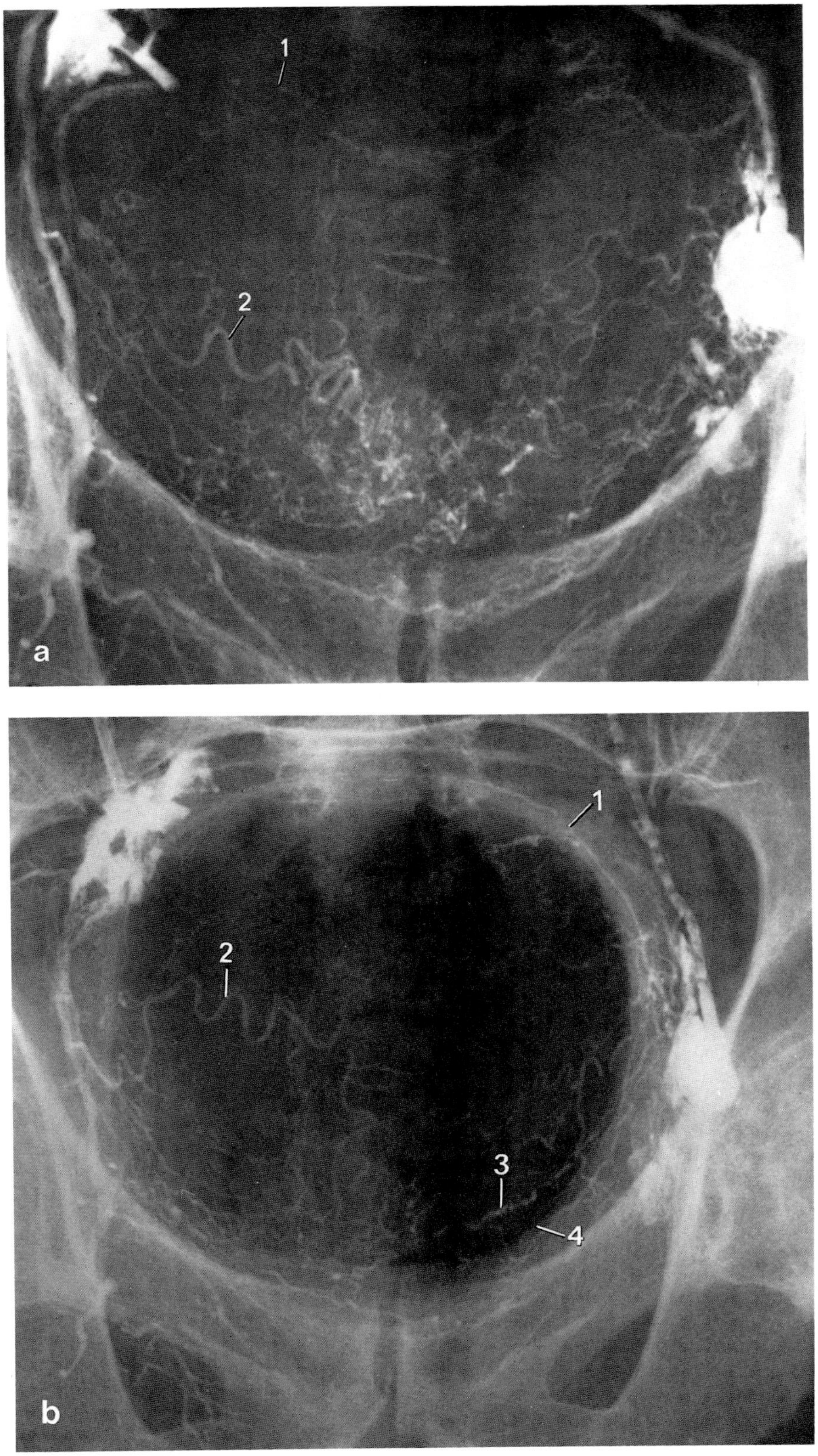

Fig. 48 a, b.
Anatomic specimen:
a empty and **b** full bladder
1 superior vesical artery
2 lateral vesical artery
3 inferior vesical artery
4 prostatic artery

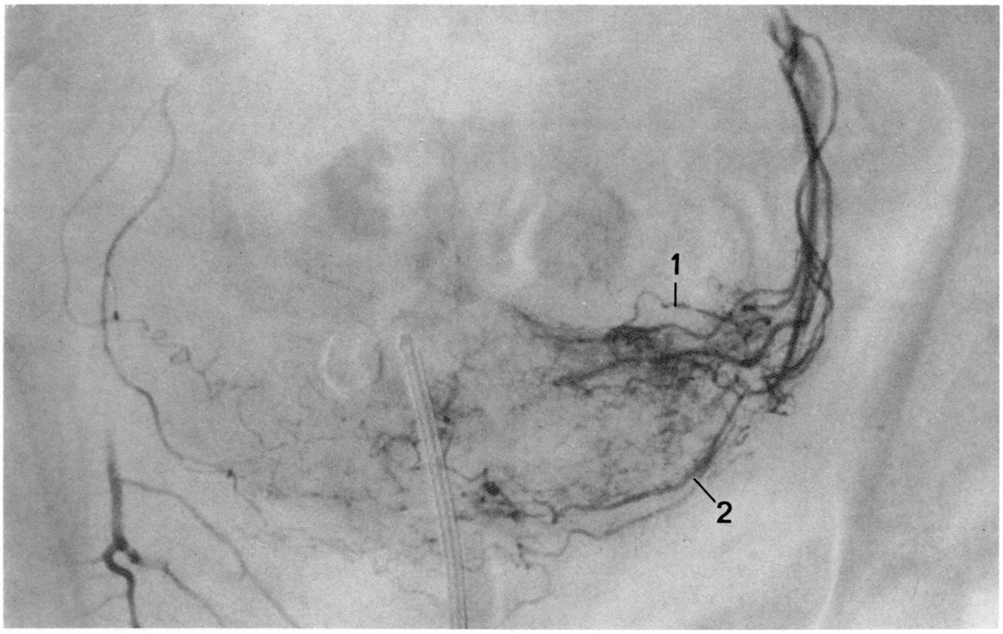

Fig. 49. Vesical arteries (empty bladder)
1 superior vesical artery
2 inferior vesical artery

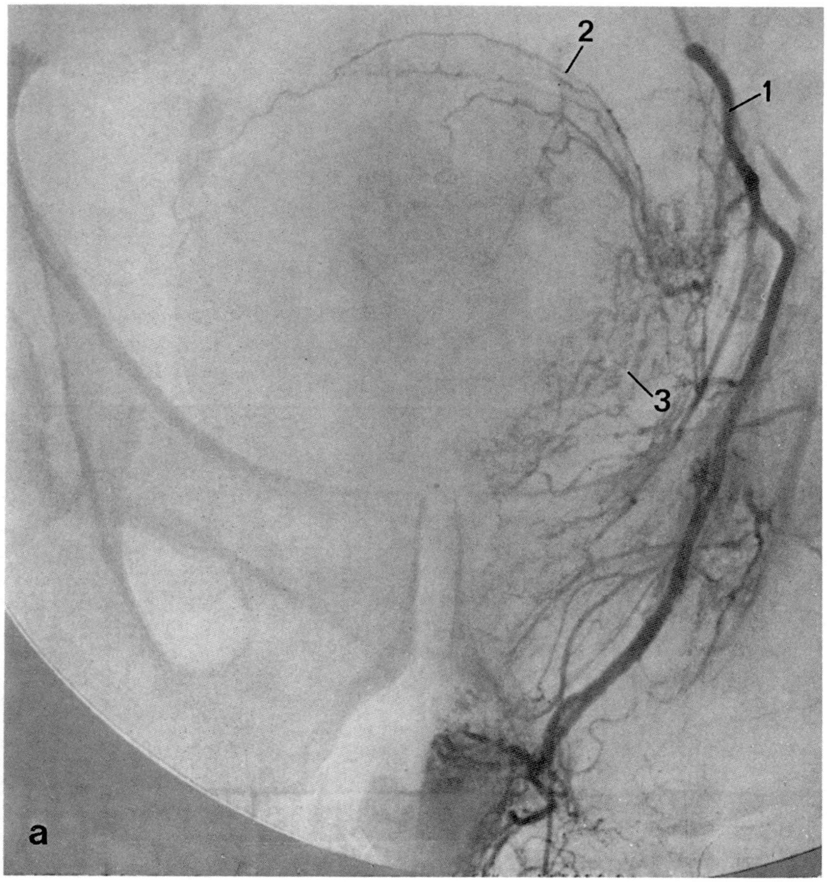

Fig. 50a. Vesical arteries (full bladder)
1 internal pudendal artery
2 superior vesical artery
3 inferior vesical artery

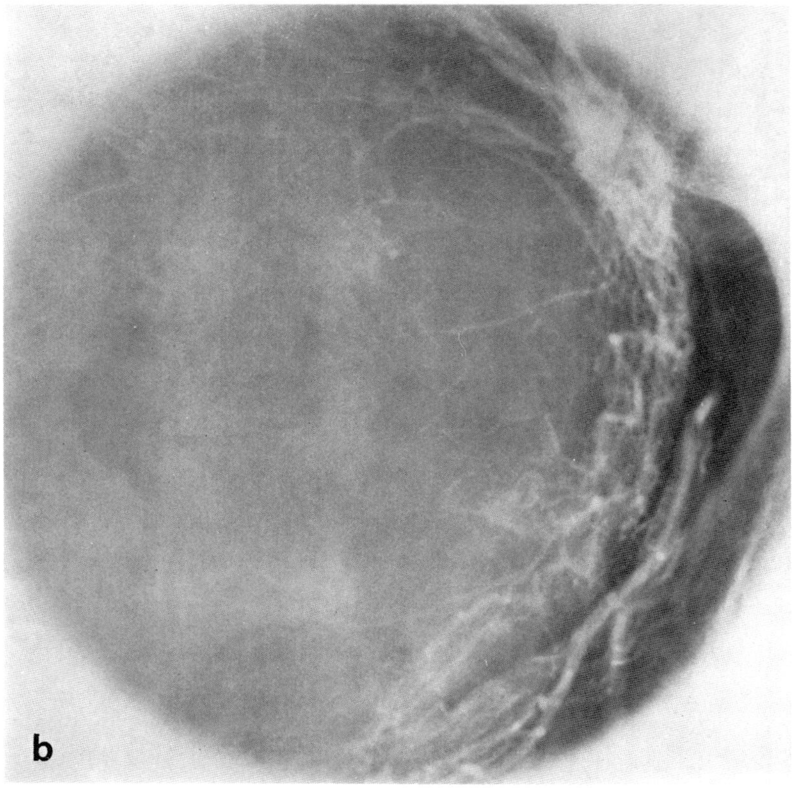

Fig. 50. b Arterial vesical network
c Anatomic specimen

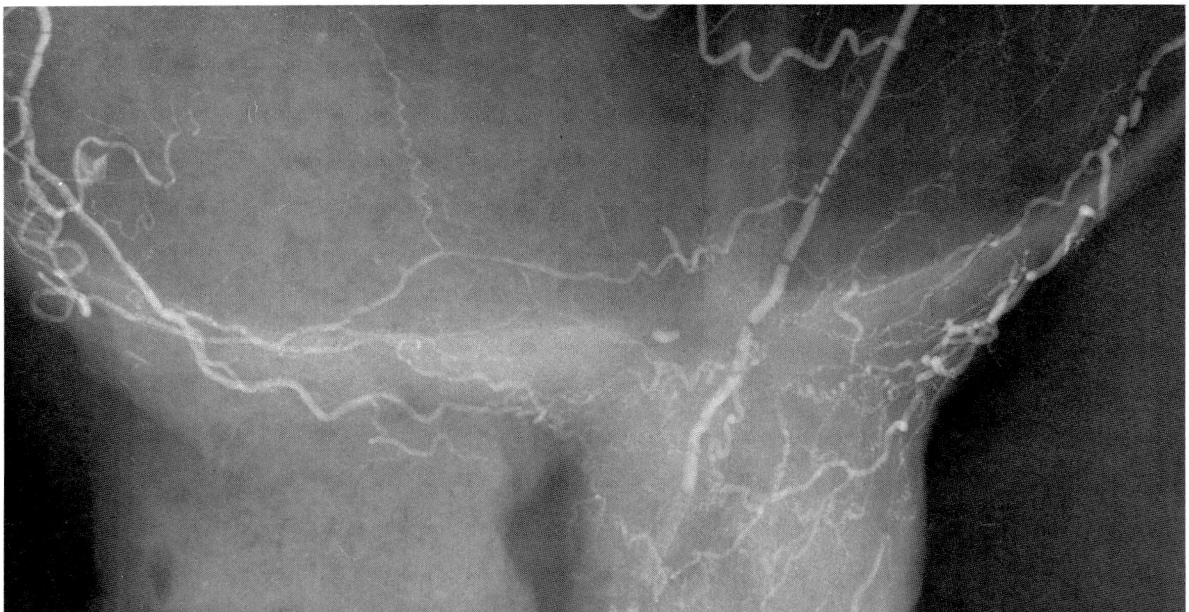

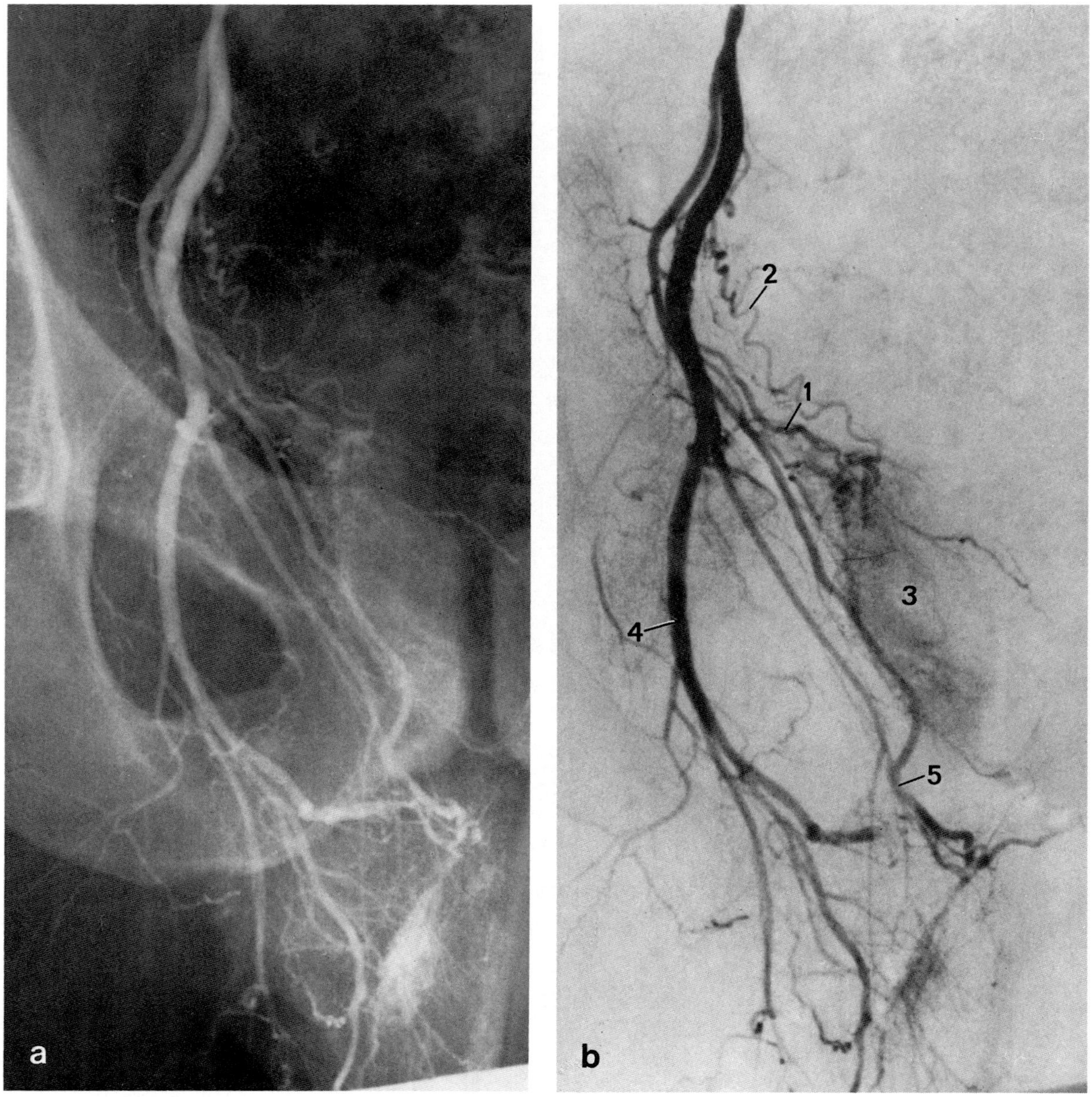

Fig. 51 a, b. Genital arteries in man
1 prostatic artery
2 vesicular artery
3 prostate
4 internal pudendal artery
5 inferior hemorrhoidal artery

The radiologic characteristics of the prostatic artery are:
a) A suprapubic, downward, medial course.
b) It divides at the lateral angle of the prostate into two or three branches.
c) Injection of the prostatic space during capillary filling.

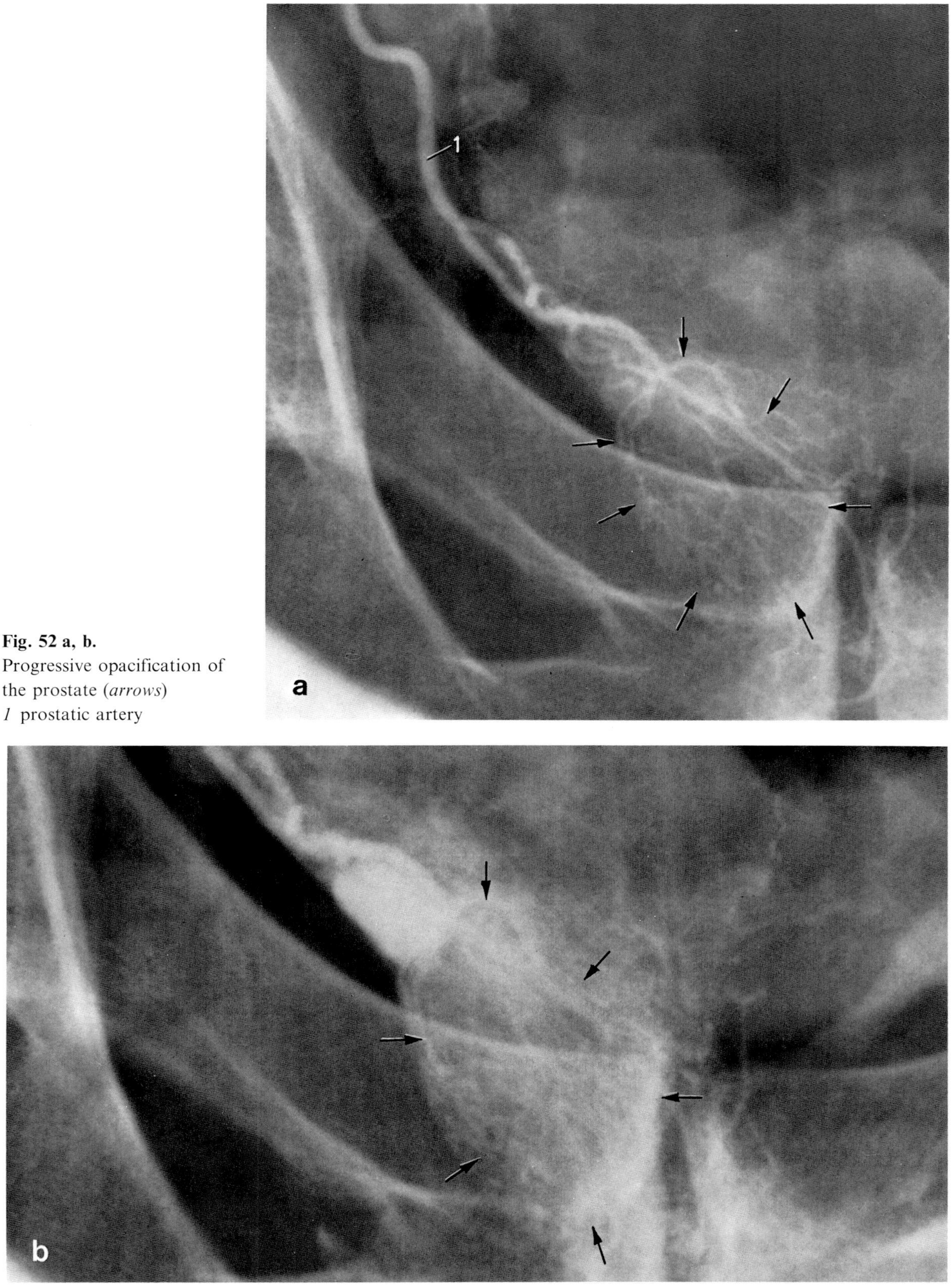

Fig. 52 a, b.
Progressive opacification of the prostate (*arrows*)
1 prostatic artery

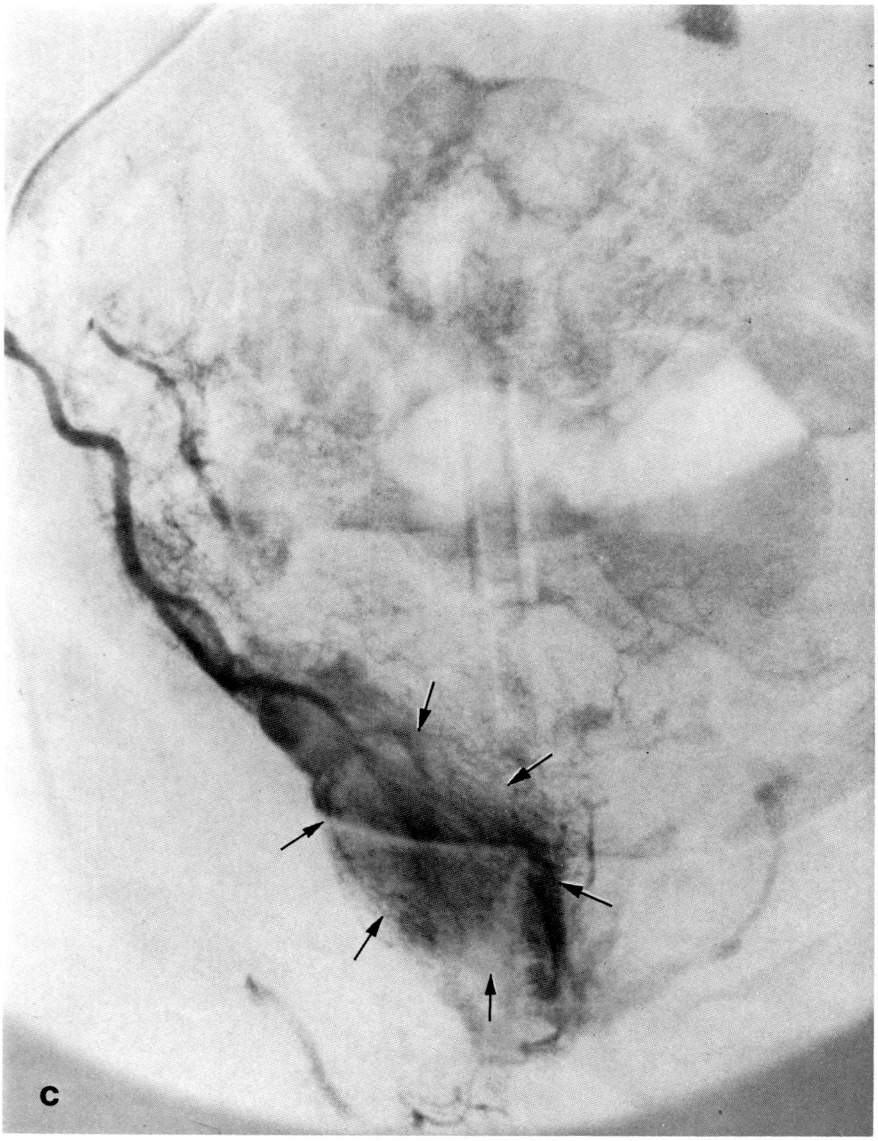

Fig. 52c. Progressive opacification of the prostate (*arrows*)

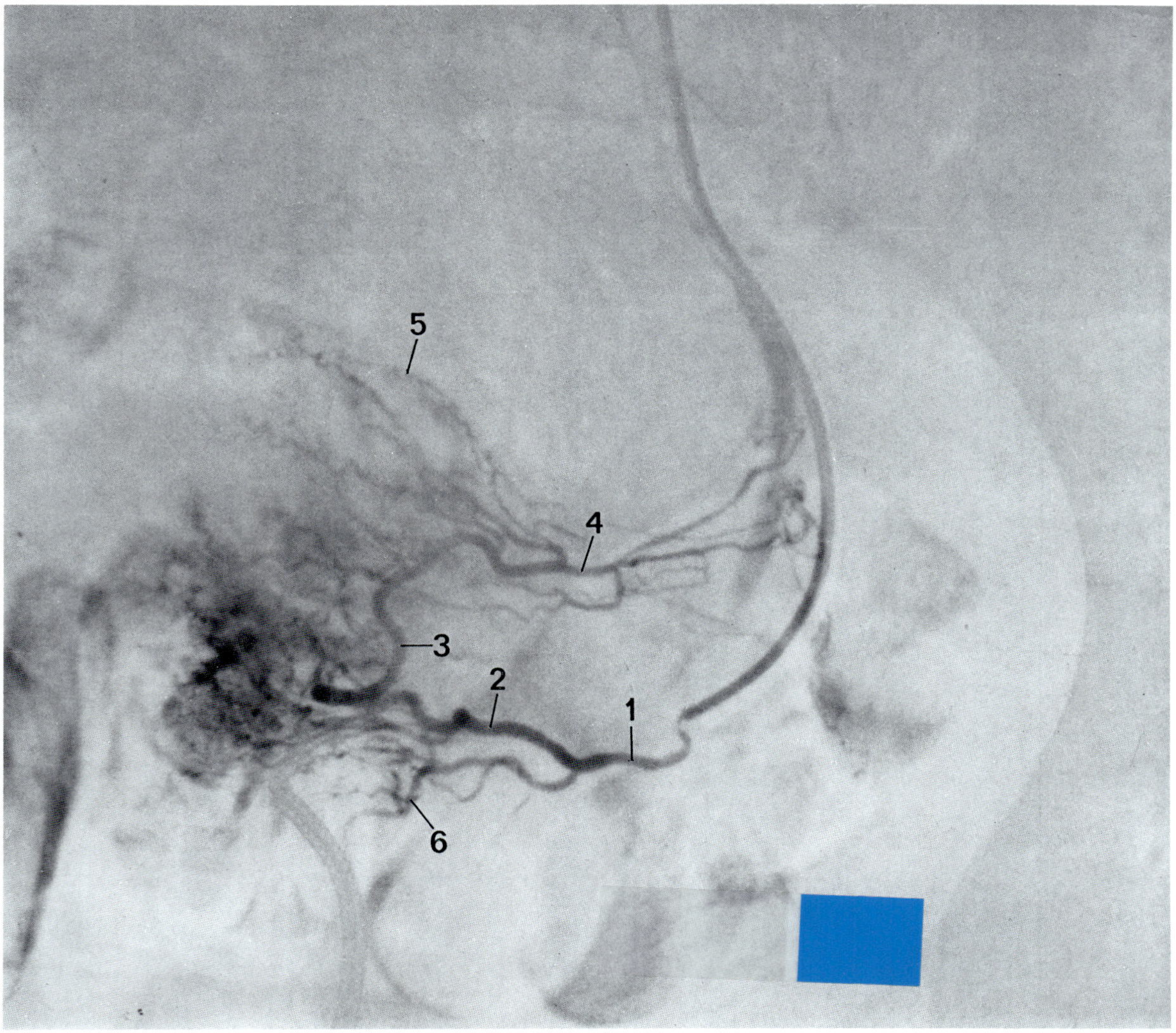

Fig. 53. Uterine artery
1 lateropelvic segment
2 mesosalpinx segment
3 laterouterine segment
4 tubal branch
5 artery for the upper surface of the uterus
6 vaginal artery

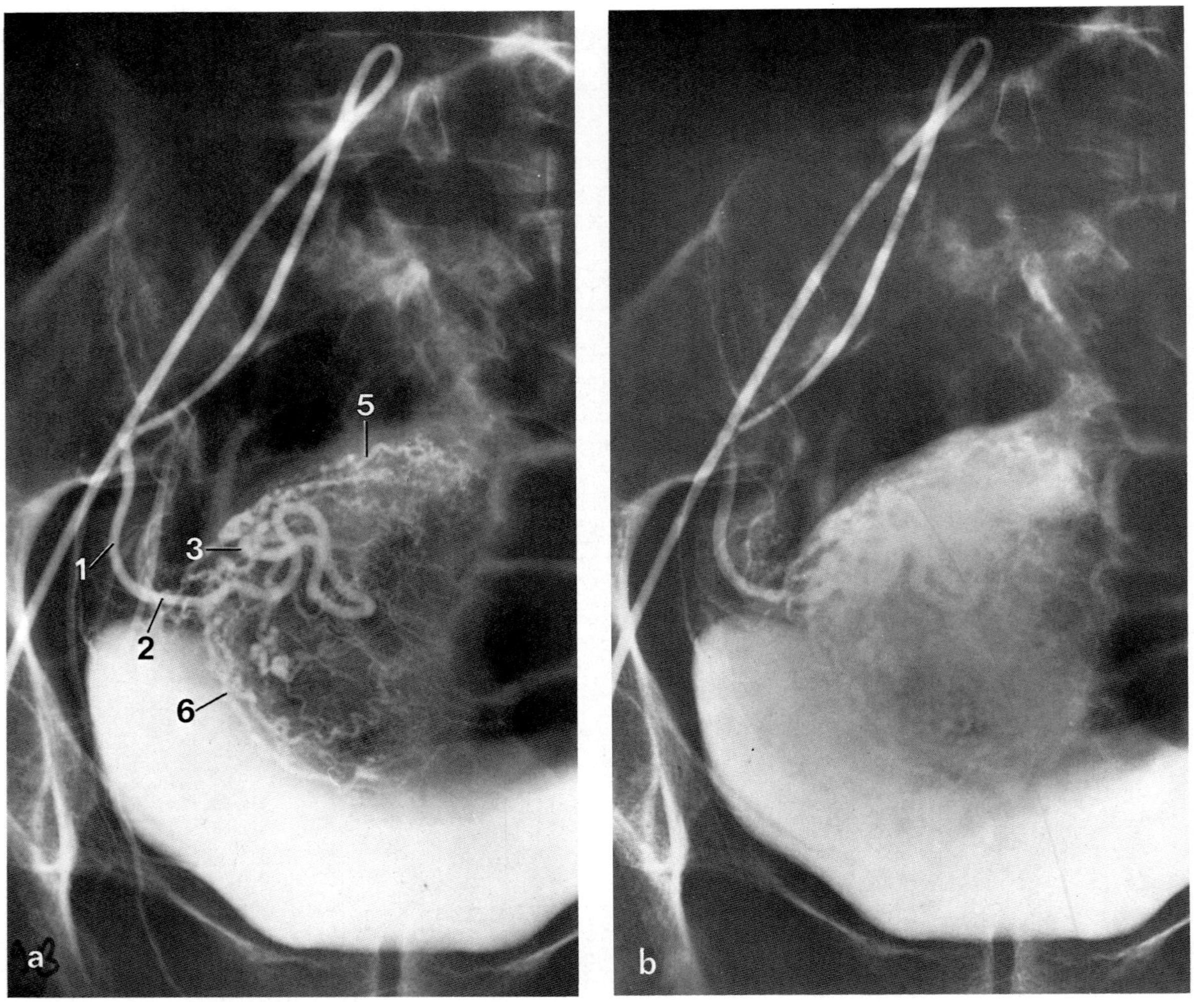

Fig. 54 a, b. Hypertrophied uterine artery (same legend as Fig. 53)

The radiologic characteristics of the uterine artery are:
a) "U"-shaped course.
b) Its ascending part gives off numerous convoluted branches that ramify horizontally.
c) Configuration variable according to uterine position.
d) Dense opacification of half of the uterus.

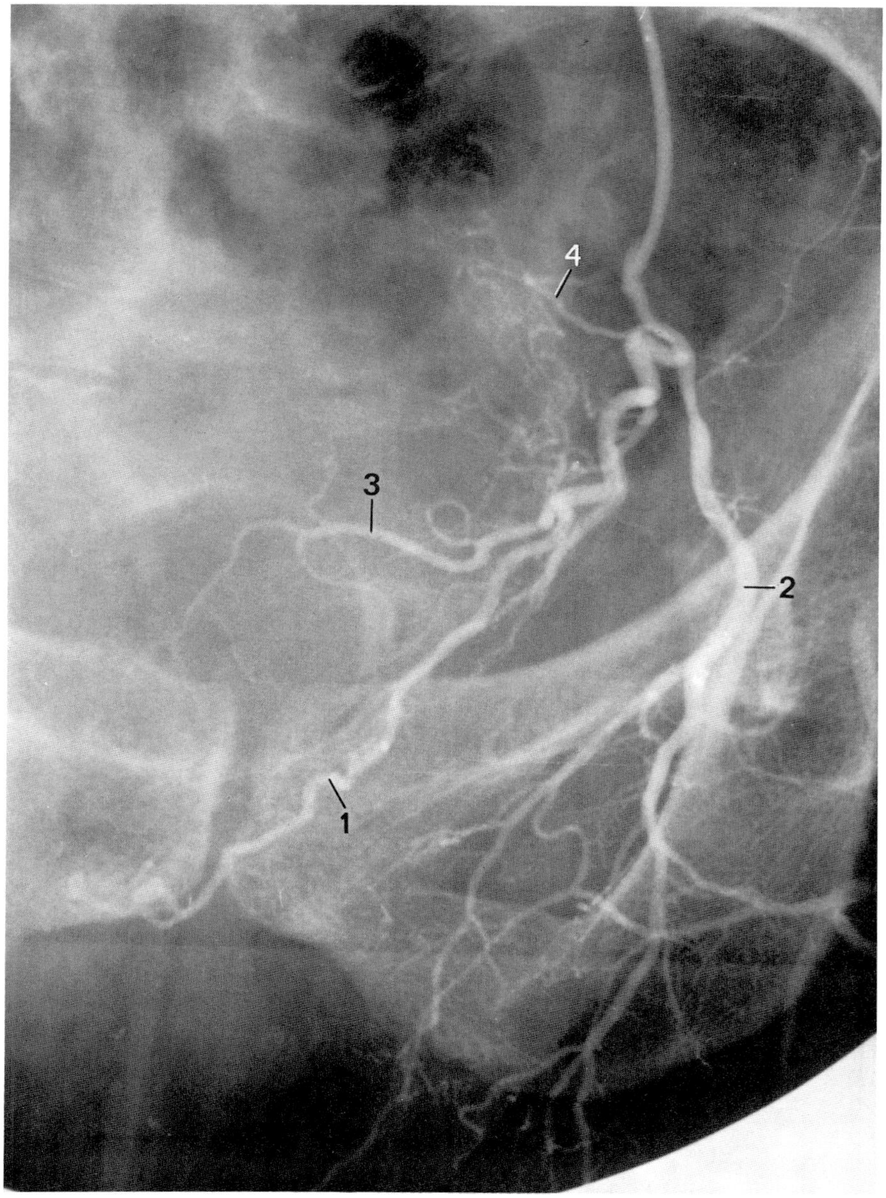

Fig. 55. Vaginal artery
1 internal pudendal artery
2 obturator artery
3 vaginal artery
4 vaginal branches

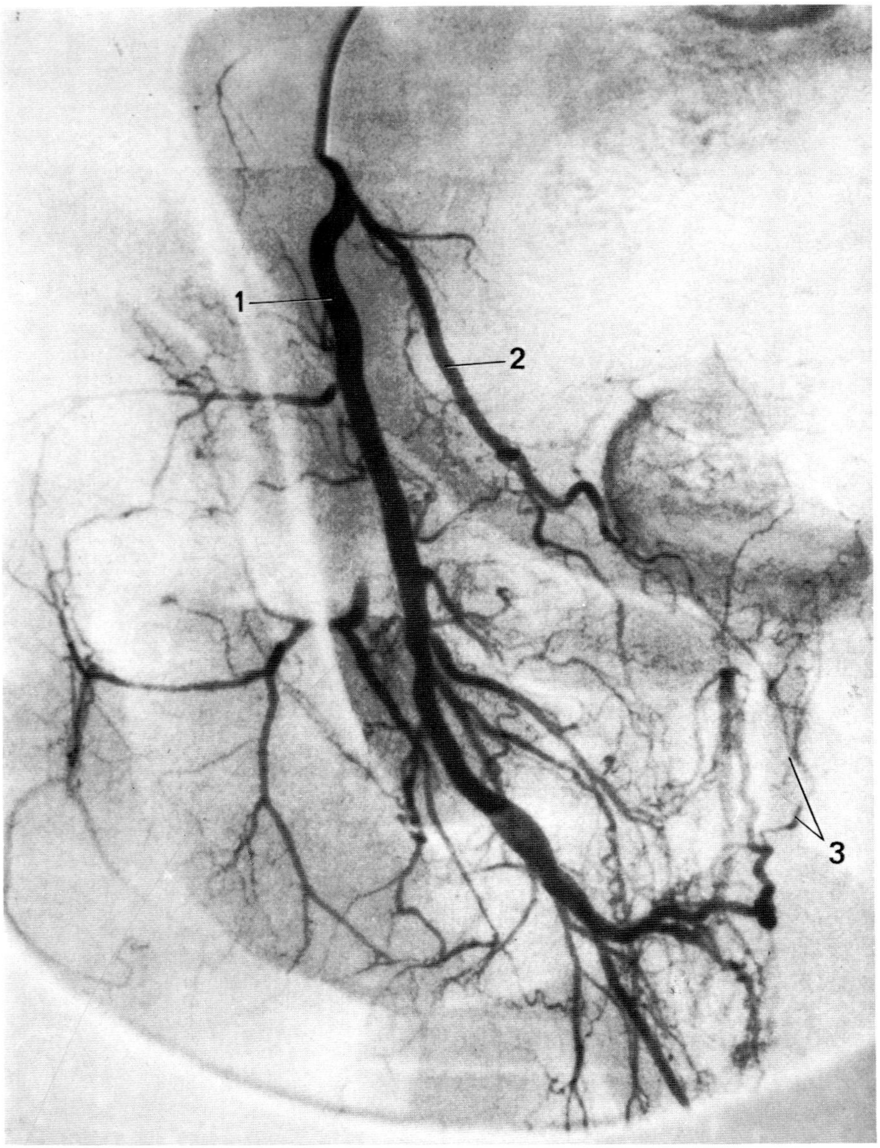

Fig. 56. Middle rectal (hemorrhoidal) artery arising from internal pudendal artery
1 internal pudendal artery
2 middle rectal artery
3 network for the anal canal

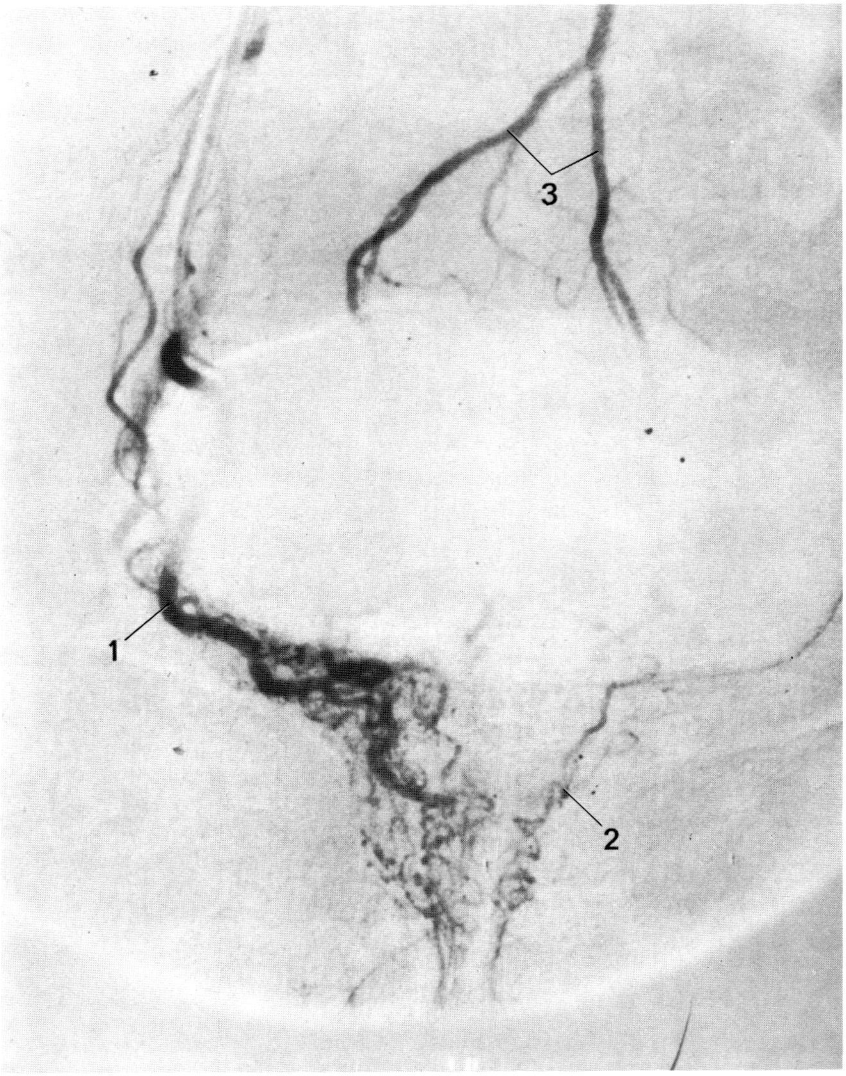

Fig. 57. Middle rectal artery (*1*), network for the anal canal (*2*), superior rectal artery (*3*)

The radiologic characteristics of the middle rectal artery are:

a) An intrapelvic downward median course.

b) It terminates behind the midpoint of the pubis in the form of a vertical vascular network.

c) Marked opacification of the inferior portion of the rectum more clearly visible following insufflation.

d) Retrograde opacification of the superior rectal artery.

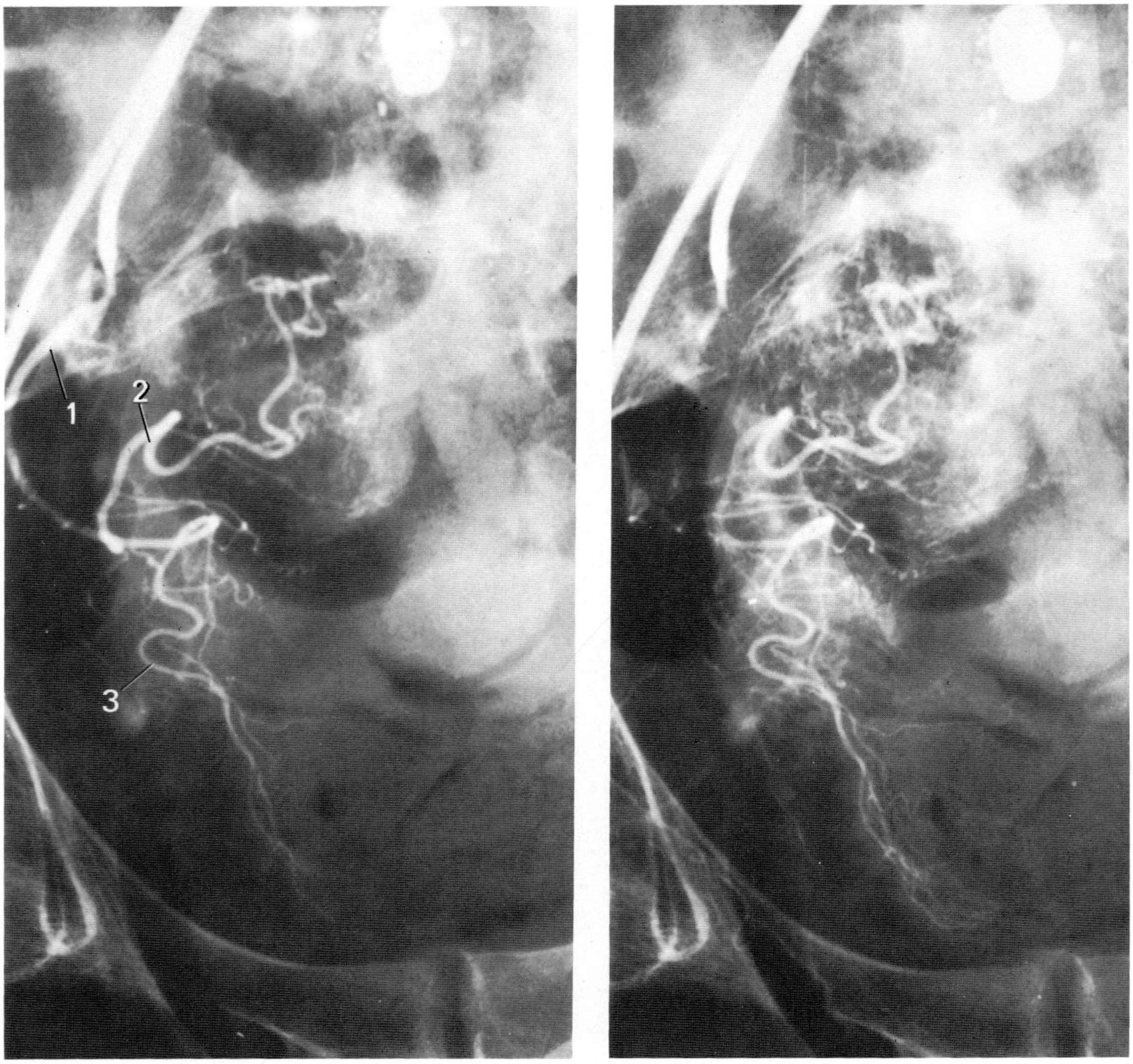

Fig. 58. Middle rectal artery (*1*) supplies all the rectum, dividing into superior (*2*) and inferior (*3*) branches

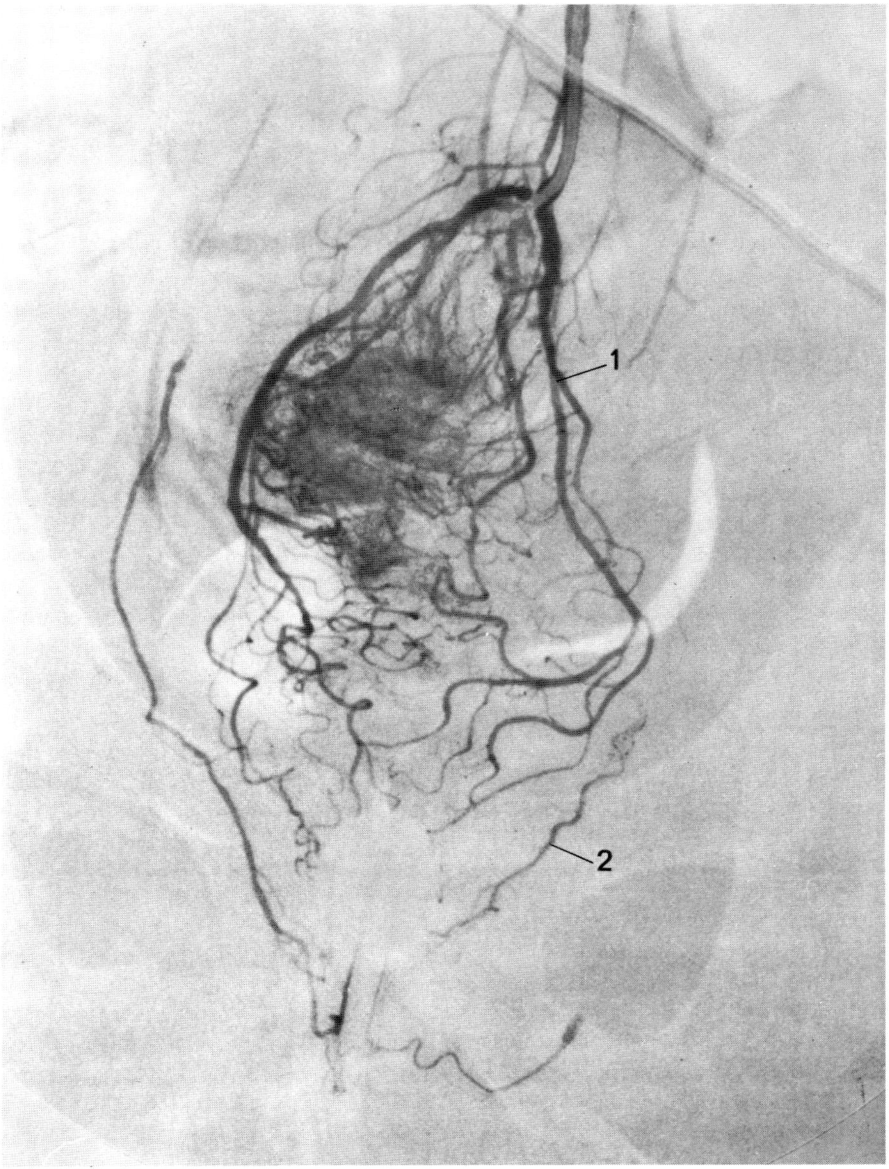

Fig. 59. Superior rectal artery (*1*): backflow into the middle rectal artery (*2*)

The radiologic characteristics of the superior rectal artery are that:

a) It is the medial branch of the inferior mesenteric artery.

b) It bifurcates and takes on a "crab claw" shape, parallel to the rectal ampulla.

c) It exhibits concomitant opacification of the inferior and middle rectal arteries.

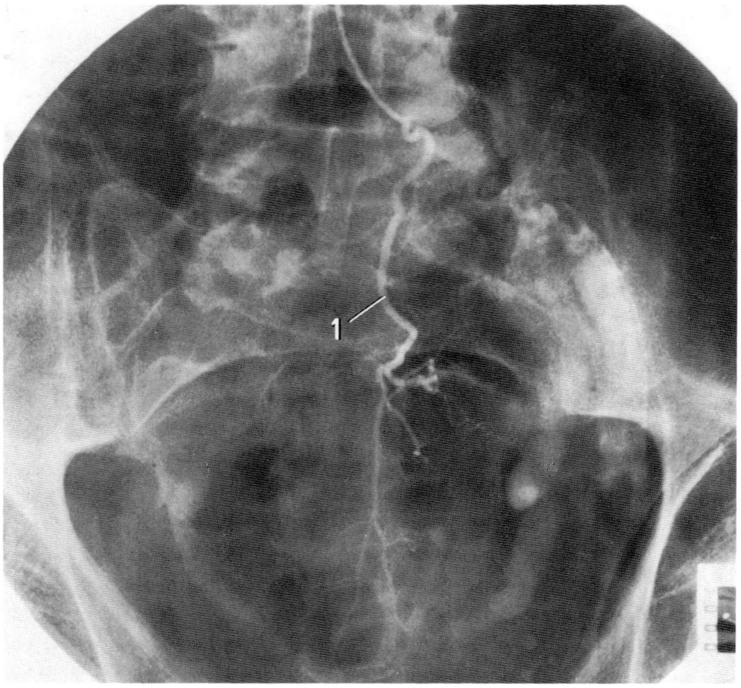

Fig. 60. Middle sacral artery (*1*) arises independently

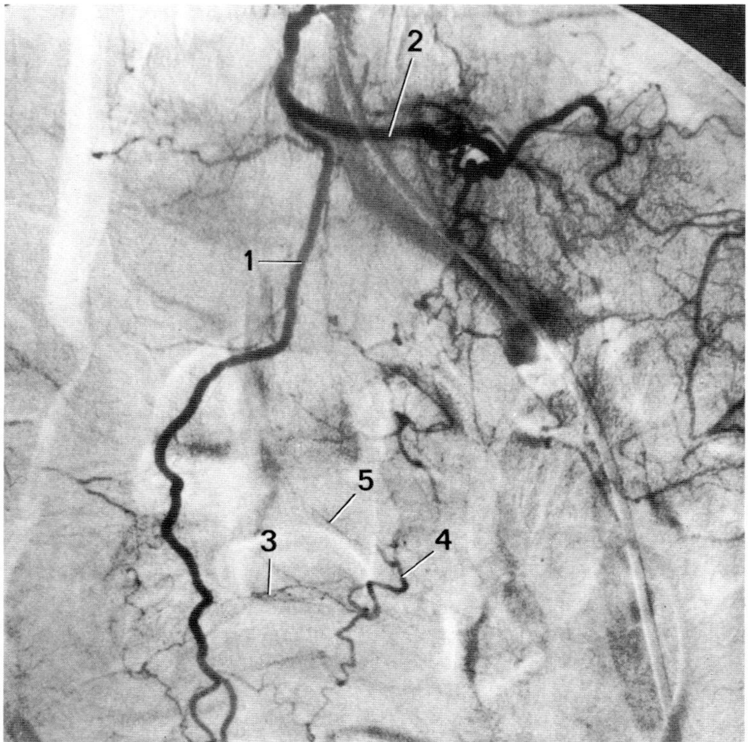

Fig. 61. Middle sacral artery (*1*) giving a voluminous fifth left lumbar artery (*2*). Anastomoses in front of the sacrum (*3*) with the lateral sacral arteries (*4*). Spinal branch (*5*)

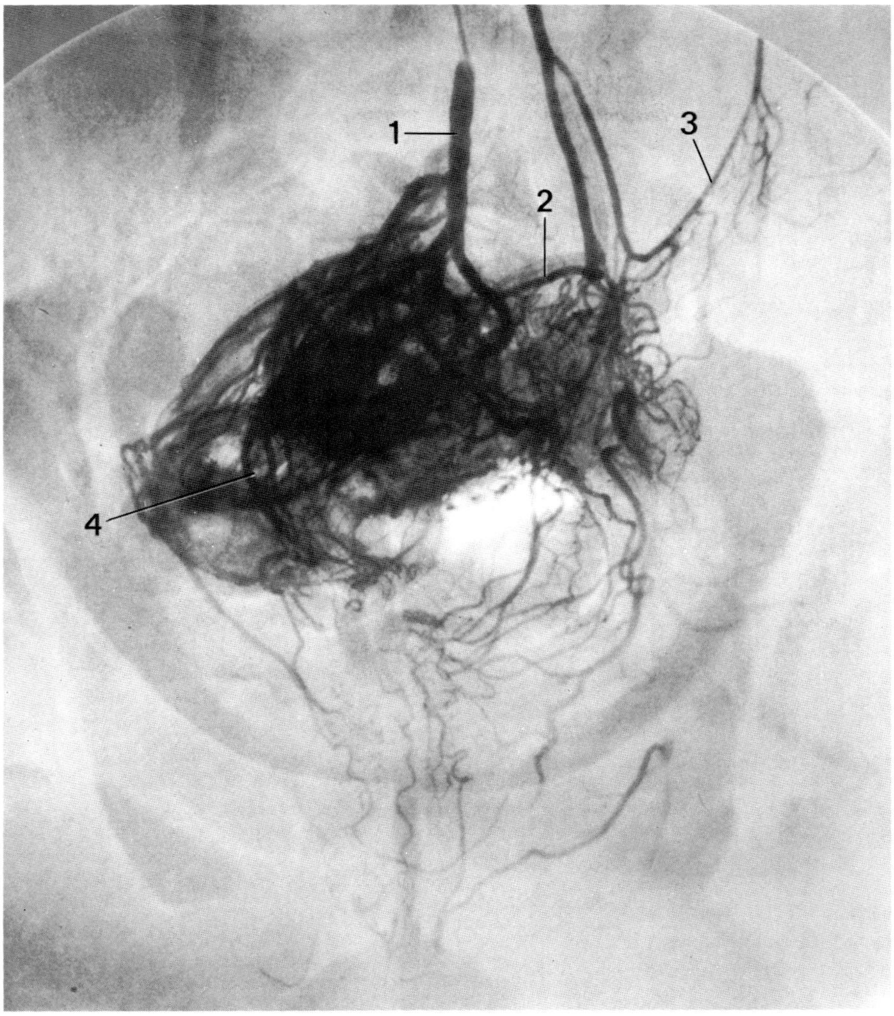

Fig. 62. Superior rectal artery (*1*), Sudeck's arch (*2*), sigmoid arteries (*3*), right lateral rectal branch (*4*)

◁ The radiologic characteristics of the middle sacral artery are:
a) Central location.
b) Vertical course along the anterior surface of the sacrum.
c) Extension to the point of the coccyx, where it anastomoses with the lateral sacral arteries.

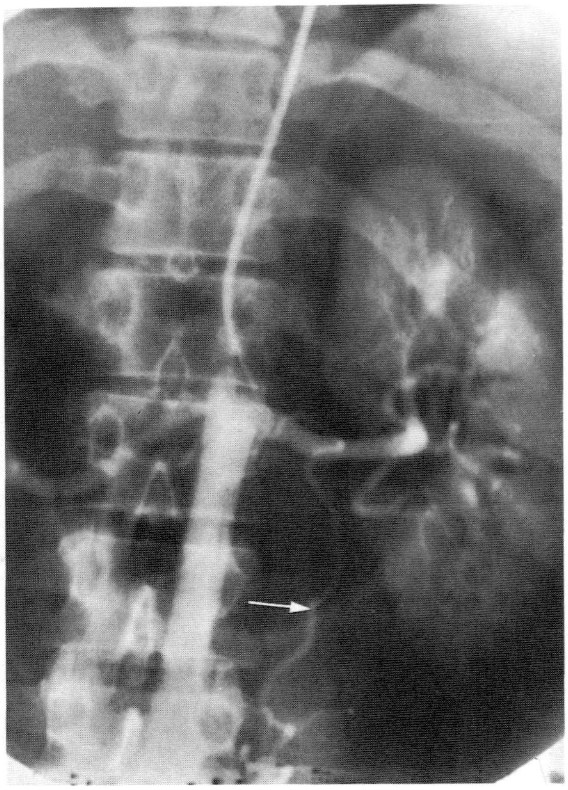

Fig. 64. Ovarian artery (*arrow*)

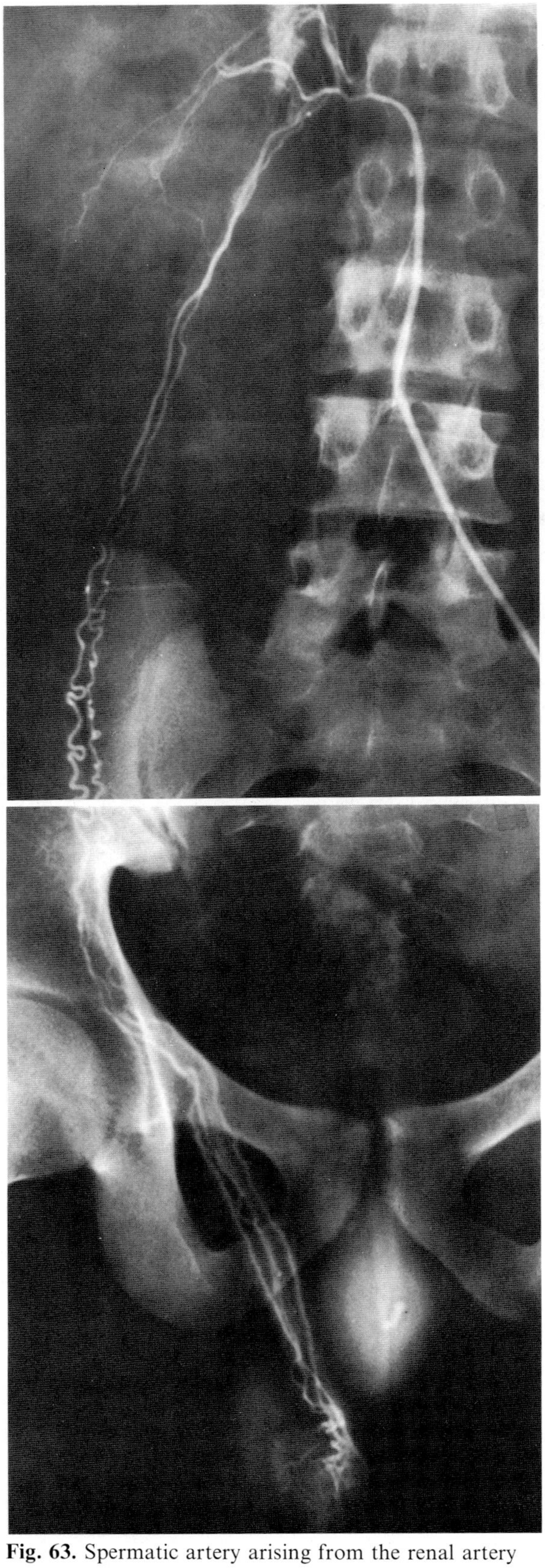

Fig. 63. Spermatic artery arising from the renal artery

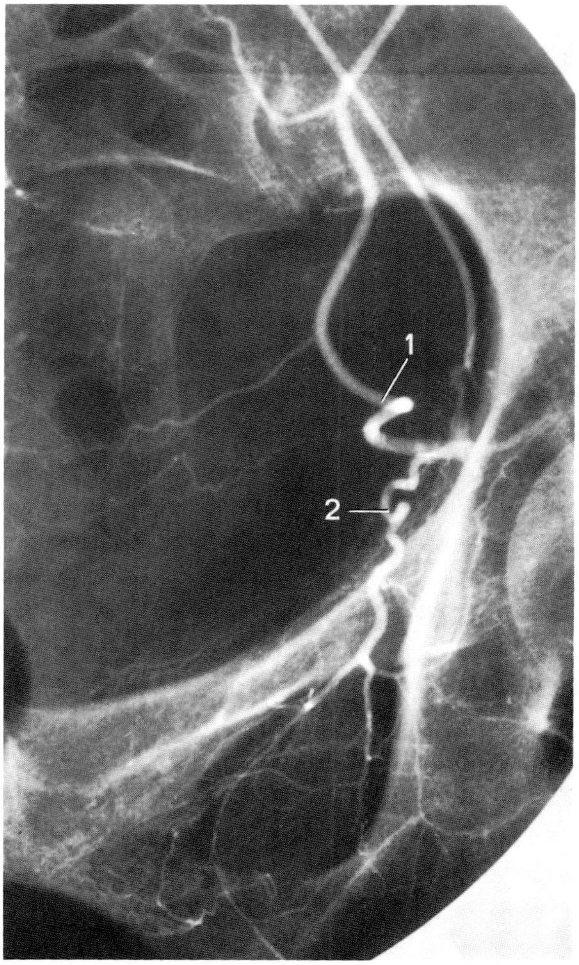

Fig. 65. Inferior epigastric artery (*1*) from which arises the obturator artery (*2*)

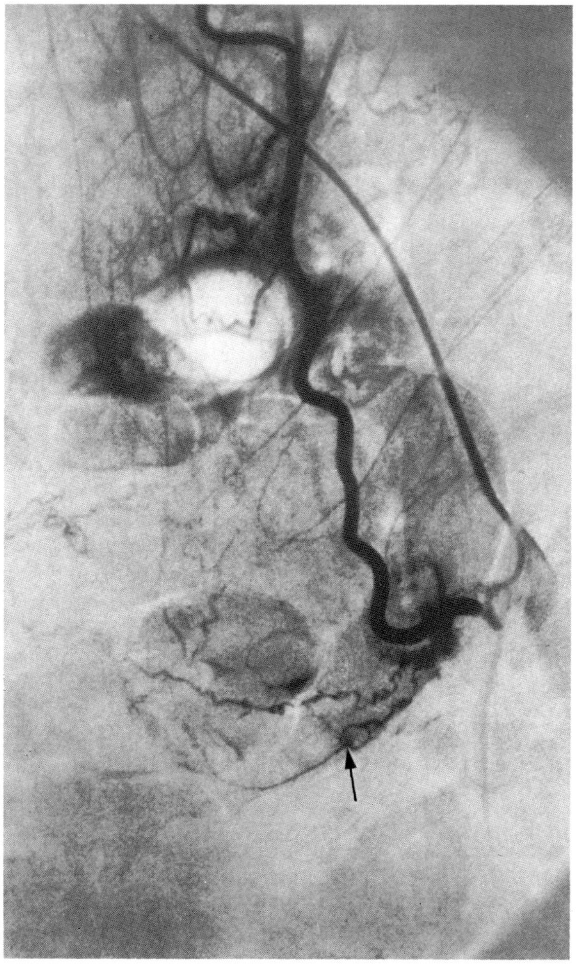

Fig. 66. Suprapubic branch of inferior epigastric artery (*arrow*)

The radiologic characteristics of the inferior epigastric artery are:
a) It arises from the external iliac artery just above the inguinal ligament.
b) Its initial segment forms an inverted arch and upward medial course.

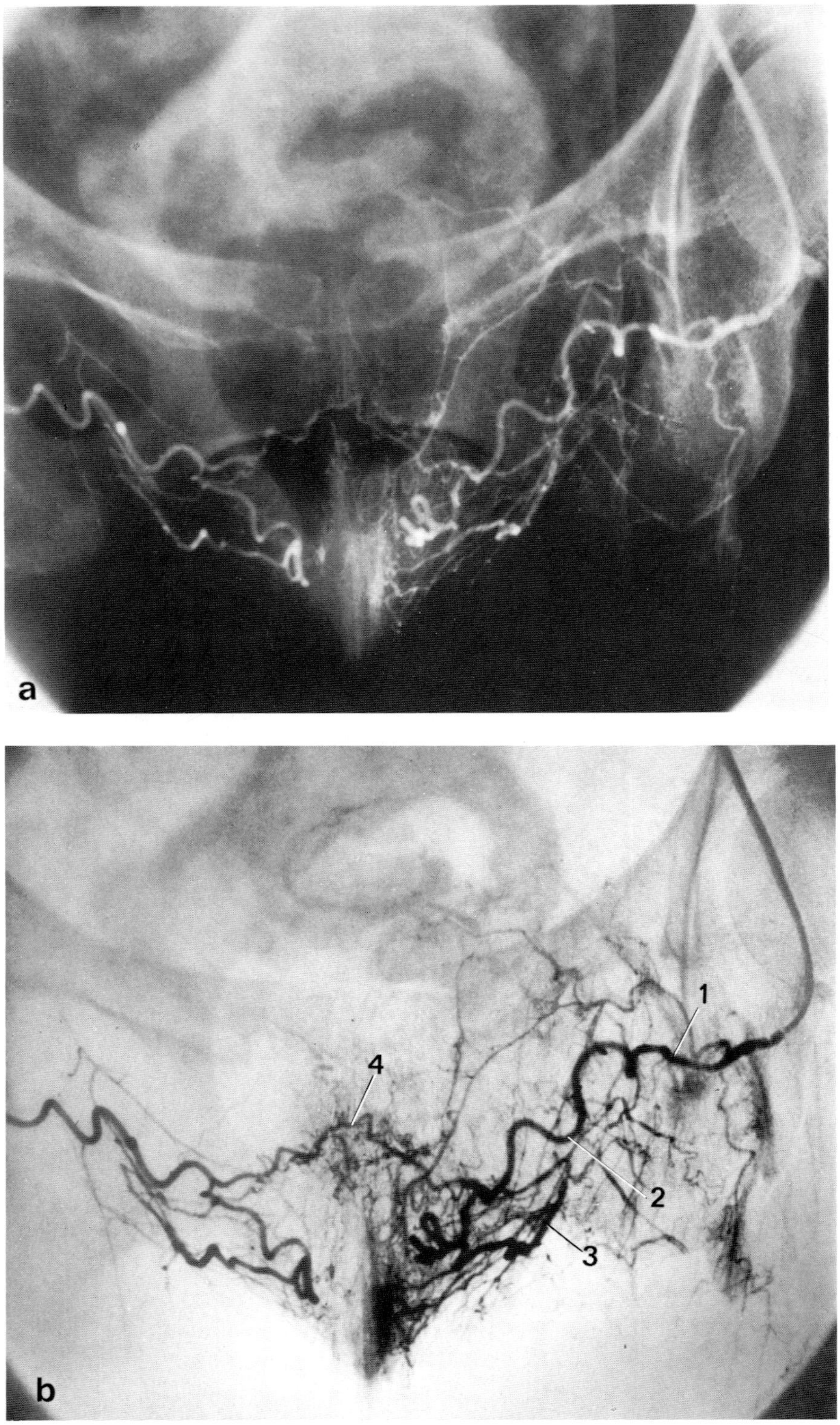

Fig. 67 a, b. External pudendal artery
1 trunk
2 superior branch
3 inferior branch
4 prepubic branch with contralateral anastomoses

3 Vascular Territories

A. Introduction

After having presented a branch-by-branch study of the blood supply of the pelvic region we shall now present an analysis of its vascular territories. For each area we shall discuss its principle blood supply as well as accessory blood supplies which can develop under pathologic circumstances. A thorough understanding of the territories is necessary in order to be able to employ therapeutic embolization.
This analysis is divided into the following three sections:

1. Blood supplies to the pelvic wall.
2. Blood supplies to the surrounding structures.
3. Blood supplies to the pelvic viscera.

B. Blood Supplies to the Pelvic Wall

I. Blood Supply to the Sacrum (Figs. 68, 69)

Blood supply to the sacrum is essentially derived from four arteries which freely anastomose along its edges, it anterior surface, and within the sacral canal:

a) The branches of the middle sacral artery, a terminal branch of the abdominal aorta, singular, and centrally placed.
b) The lateral sacral arteries, which usually number from two to four and arise from the trunk of the internal iliac artery or from one of its branches.
c) The iliolumbar artery supplies by means of its lumbar division the first sacral segment and its wing.

Lastly, certain branches can furnish an accessory blood supply to the sacrum: the superior and middle rectal arteries, the inferior and superior gluteal arteries.

II. Blood Supply to the Hip Bone (Fig. 70)

Since the hip bone receives numerous small branches arising from neighboring arteries, its blood supply is rather intricate.
The ilium receives small branches from the iliolumbar, superior gluteal, deep circumflex iliac, and lumbar arteries. The latter two arteries also supply the iliac crest.
The ischium receives vessels from the internal pudendal artery and small branches from the inferior gluteal artery. The acetabulum is supplied by the acetabular artery, a branch of the obturator artery, which is easily identifiable during arteriography by its characteristic course. The rami of ischium and pubis are supplied by branches of the obturator artery.
The pubis receives vessels from the internal pudendal artery, principally in the form of small periostic arteries subject to a great deal of variation.

III. Blood Supply to the Pelvic Floor (Fig. 71)

A distinction is made between the blood supply to the midline and to the lateral portions.
The midline area is supplied by branches of the internal pudendal, vaginal (in the female), and inferior hemorrhoidal arteries.

The lateral portions receive vessels from the following three arteries:

a) The obturator artery: gives off many small branches along the lateral brim of the pelvis which supply the levator muscles.
b) Branches of the inferior gluteal artery which furnish the major portion of the blood supply to the levator muscles.
c) The middle sacral and lateral sacral arteries.

C. Blood Supplies to the Extrapelvic Structures

Schematically speaking, we can identify pedicles which supply the gluteal region, the posteroproximal part of the thigh, the obturator region, the perineal area, and the external genitalia in the male.

I. Gluteal Region (Fig. 72)

This area is supplied by the superior gluteal artery. The inferior gluteal artery usually supplies the lower quarter of this region. The superficial branches of the superior gluteal artery provide an anastomotic link with the inferior gluteal artery.
Other arteries, however, can participate to a lesser degree in the blood supply of this area. In cases of arterial obstruction these arteries play a major role in feeding this area. They comprise:

a) The fourth lumbar artery, which supplies the posterior wall of the abdomen and the iliac crest.
b) The deep circumflex iliac and iliolumbar arteries, which supply the iliac fossa. Some branches may pass around the iliac wing and anastomose with branches of the superior gluteal artery.
c) The lateral circumflex artery, which arises from the deep femoral artery. This artery anastomoses with small branches of the inferior gluteal artery and supplies the lower portion of the gluteal region.
d) The medial circumflex artery can in cases supply the lateral part of the gluteal region.

II. Posteroproximal Part of the Thigh (Fig. 73)

The inferior gluteal artery supplies the teguments, and the medial femoral circumflex artery supplies the hip joint. In addition, the superior gluteal artery, branches of the obturator artery, and the initial perforating arteries of the deep femoral artery contribute to a lesser degree to the blood supply of this area. The role which the anastomotic network of the inferior gluteal artery plays in forming a collateral system for the inferior extremity in cases of arteriosclerotic occlusions of the iliofemoral arterial axis should be noted; nor should its role in arteriovenous malformations of the root of the lower extremity be overlooked.

III. Obturator Region (Fig. 74)

The deep part of this area is supplied by the obturator and inferior epigastric arteries. These two arteries clearly anastomose, which explains the possibility that the obturator artery can arise from the arch of the epigastric artery. They participate equally in the blood supply of this region, but on occasion the obturator takes on a preponderant role.
The superficial part is supplied by the external pudendal artery, which runs across the obturator region and terminates in the perineal region. In addition, the internal pudendal artery gives off branches to this area:

a) Small branches which pass via the obturator foramen.
b) Branches of the perineal artery.

IV. Perineal Area (Fig. 75)

This area is supplied by the internal and external pudendal arteries.

- By means of its perineal and inferior hemorrhoidal branches the internal pudendal artery supplies the anal canal and the central and anterior portions of the perineum. The external pudendal artery gives off vessels to the portion of the perineum in front of the root of the penis in the male and the urinary meatus in the female. The extensive anastomotic network between the two arterial systems should be emphasized and is readily demonstrated by the fact that injection of the internal pudendal artery opacifies the entire perineal region. In addition, the obturator artery contributes to the blood supply of this area by means of its anastomoses with the internal or external pudendal arteries.

V. External Genitalia in the Male

a) The penis is supplied in its totality by the terminal branches of the internal pudendal artery, which anastomose with their fellow arteries. Under pathologic circumstances the external pudendal artery contributes to the blood supply of this area by means of the anastomoses with the internal pudendal artery at the base of the penis.

b) The scrotum has a double blood supply coming from the external pudendal artery, branches of the femoral artery, and the perineal artery, itself a branch of the internal pudendal artery. These branches anastomose in the subcutaneous tissues of the scrotum.
The deep layers are supplied by the external spermatic artery, which arises from the epigastric artery. It anastomoses with the internal spermatic and deferential arteries.

c) The testicle is supplied by the internal spermatic artery, which arises from the aorta at the L-2 level, and by the deferential artery, which supplies the ductus deferens.

D. Blood Supplies to the Pelvic Viscera

I. Bladder (Fig. 76)

The blood supply to the bladder comes from two principle pedicles: the superior vesical artery and the inferior vesical artery, which together supply it in its entirety. These arteries may arise in variable fashion from the anterior division of the hypogastric artery (either by a common trunk or from an umbilical artery which gives off the superior vesical artery) or from a genitovesical artery which gives off the inferior vesical artery and the genital artery (vaginal in the female and prostatic in the male).
In addition the internal pudendal artery gives off thin vesical branches which supply the trigone. In both the male and female the middle rectal and the uterine arteries can contribute to the blood supply of the bladder.

II. Rectum (Fig. 77)

The blood supply of the rectum comes from three arteries:

a) The superior rectal artery, which supplies the rectal ampulla.

b) The middle artery, which supplies the lower portion of the ampulla and the anal canal and, in certain cases, the rectum in its entirety.

c) The inferior rectal artery, which arises from the internal pudendal artery and supplies the anal margin.
Small branches of the uterine, vesical, and sacral arteries can form a collateral network which is minimal except in cases of local neoplastic process.

III. Female Genital Organs (Fig. 78)

1. Uterus

The uterus, including its annexes, is supplied by the uterine artery and its branches. A non-negligible contribution is made by the ovarian artery, a branch of the abdominal aorta. On the other hand, a funicular branch of the ovarian artery which accompanies the round ligament plays a very small role in the blood supply of the female genital organs.

2. Vagina

The superior portion of the vagina has a rich blood supply derived from the vaginal branch of the uterine artery; its middle portion is supplied by a vaginal branch of the inferior vesical artery, and its lower portion is supplied by the internal pudendal artery.
In addition, small branches can arise from the superior and middle rectal arteries.

IV. Accessory Male Genital Organs (Fig. 79)

The prostate, the seminal vesicles, and the vas deferens are principally supplied by the deferential and prostatic arteries. It should be noted that unlike other centrally located organs there are no anastomoses between fellow left and right prostatic arteries because of the presence of the raphe.
These organs are also supplied by branches of arteries to the neighboring organs (middle and inferior rectal, internal pudendal, and inferior vesical arteries).

	Main supply	Acessory supply
Sacral region (Fig. 1)	– Lateral sacral a. – Medial sacral a.	– Inferior gluteal a. – Superior gluteal a. – Rectal a. – Opposite sacral lateral a. – 5th lumbar a. – Ilio-Lumbar a.
Iliac bone (Fig. 2) Iliac ala	– Ilio lumbar a. – 4th lumbar a. – Obturator a. – Sup. gluteal a. – Deep circumflex iliac a.	
Acetabulum	– Obturator a. – Internal pudendal a. – Sup. gluteal a.	
Ischio pubic branch	– Obturator a. – Internal pudendal a.	
Pelvic floor (Fig. 3)	– Inf. lateral sacral a. – Inf. gluteal a. – Obturator a. – Sup. gluteal a. – Internal pudendal a.	– Middle rectal a. – Genito vesical a.
Gluteal region (Fig. 4)	– Superior gluteal a. – Inferior gluteal a.	– 4th lumbar a. – Ilio lumbar a. – Deep circumflex iliac a. – Lateral femoral circumflex a.
Posterior face of the tigh (Fig. 5)	– Inferior gluteal a. – Medial femoral circumflex a.	– Superior gluteal a. – Obturator a. – Lateral femoral circumflex a. – Perforating a.
Obturator region (Fig. 6)	– Obturator a. – Inferior epigastric a. – External pudendal a.	– Internal pudendal a. – Inferior gluteal a. – Medial femoral circumflex a.
Perineal region (Fig. 7)	– Internal pudendal a. – Middle rectal a. – External pudendal a.	– Obturator a. – Medial femoral circumflex a.
O.G.E External hali genitalia	– Inferior epigastric a. – Internal pudendal a. – External pudendal a. – Deferential a.	
Iliac fossa (Fig. 9)	– Ilio lumbar a. – Deep circumflex iliac a.	– Sup. gluteal a. – Obturator a.
Bladder (Fig. 10)	– Sup. vesical a. – Inf. vesical a.	– Internal pudendal a. – Prostatic a. – Vaginal a.
Rectum (Fig. 11)	– Sup. rectal a. – Middle rectal a. – Internal pudendal a.	
Uterus	– Uterine a. – Ovarian a. – Vaginal a.	– A. of round ligament of uterus
Vagin (Fig. 12)	– Long vaginal	– Middle rectal a. – Perineal branches of internal pudendal a.
Prostatic gland, vesicular seminales (Fig. 13)	– Prostatic a. – Vesicular a.	– Internal pudendal a.

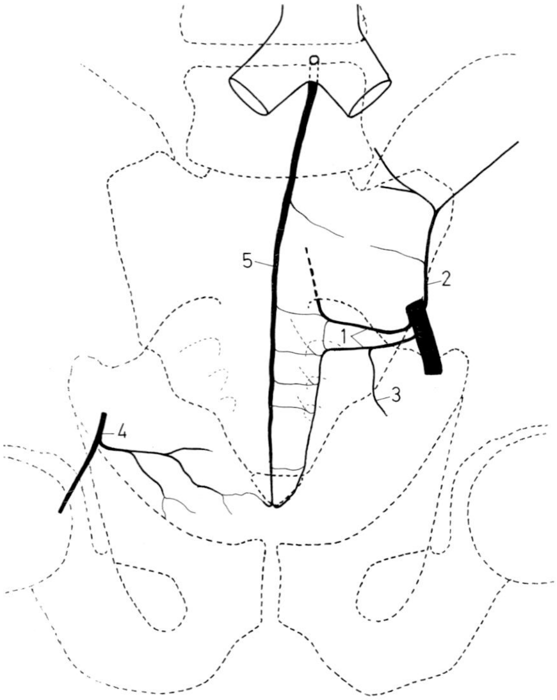

◁ **Fig. 68.** Blood supply of the sacrum
1 lateral sacral artery
2 iliolumbar artery
3 artery of the piriform muscle
4 internal branch of the inferior gluteal artery
5 medial sacral artery

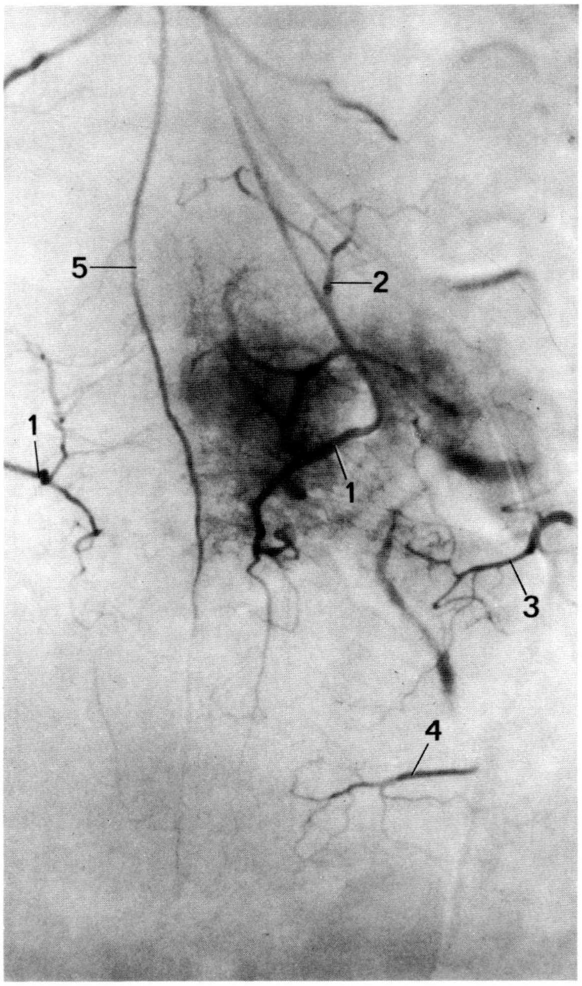

Fig. 69. Blood supply of the sacrum and the pelvic floor (same legend as Fig. 68)

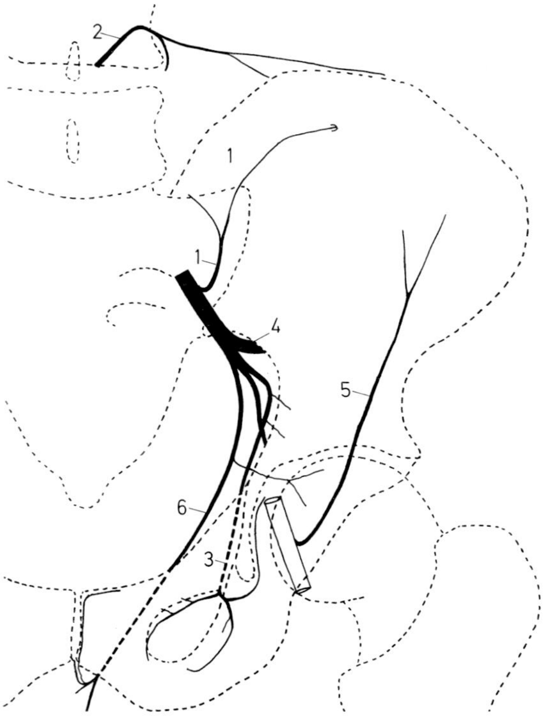

Fig. 70. Blood supply of the iliac bone
1 iliolumbar artery
2 fourth lumbar artery
3 obturator artery
4 superior gluteal artery
5 deep circumflex iliac artery
6 internal pudendal artery

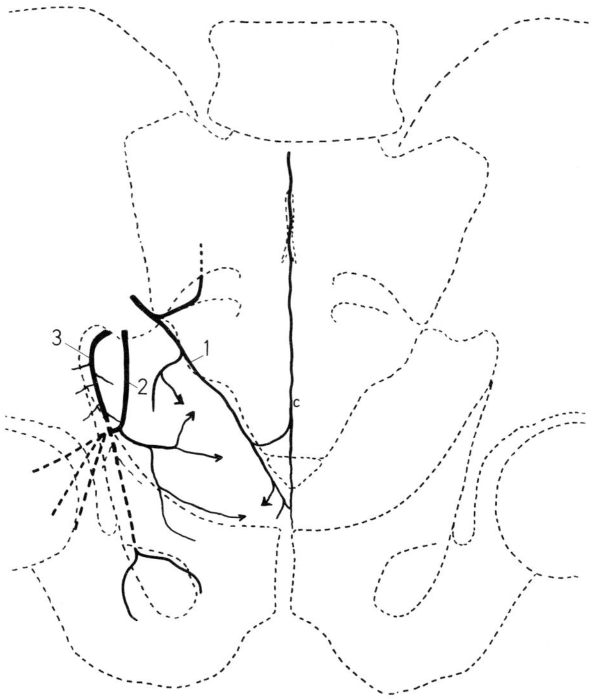

Fig. 71. Blood supply for the pelvic floor
1 lateral sacral artery
2 inferior gluteal artery
3 obturator artery

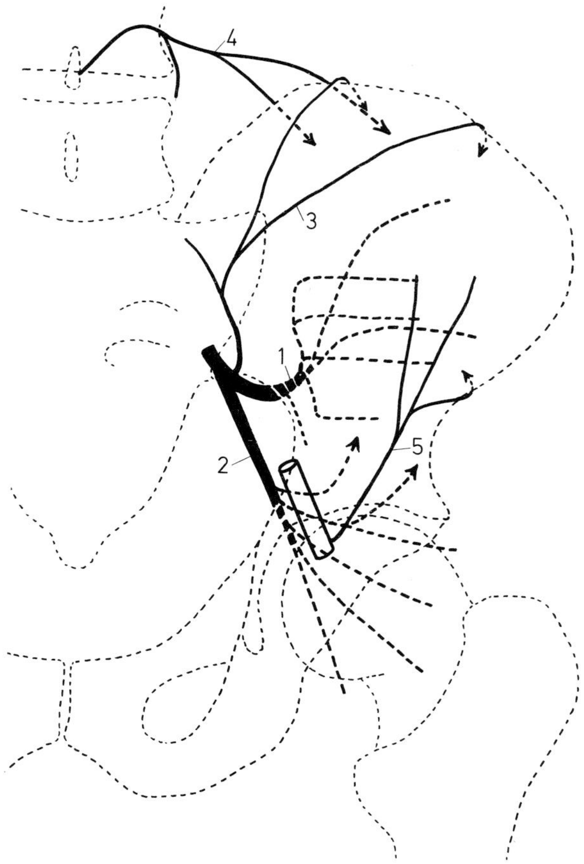

Fig. 72. Blood supply of the gluteal region
1 superior gluteal artery
2 inferior gluteal artery
3 iliolumbar artery
4 fourth lumbar artery
5 deep circumflex artery

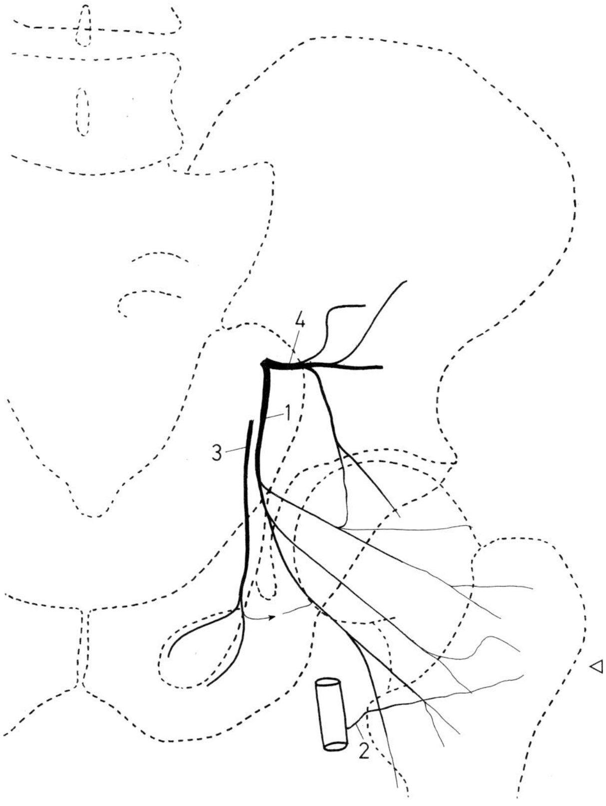

◁ **Fig. 73.** Blood supply of the posterior part of the thigh
1 inferior gluteal artery
2 circumflex femoral artery
3 obturator artery
4 superior gluteal artery

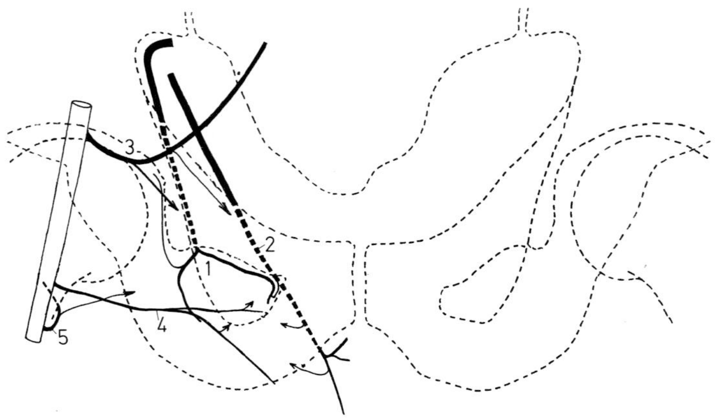

Fig. 74. Blood supply of the obturator region
1 obturator artery
2 internal pudendal artery
3 inferior epigastric artery
4 external pudendal artery
5 deep circumflex femoral artery

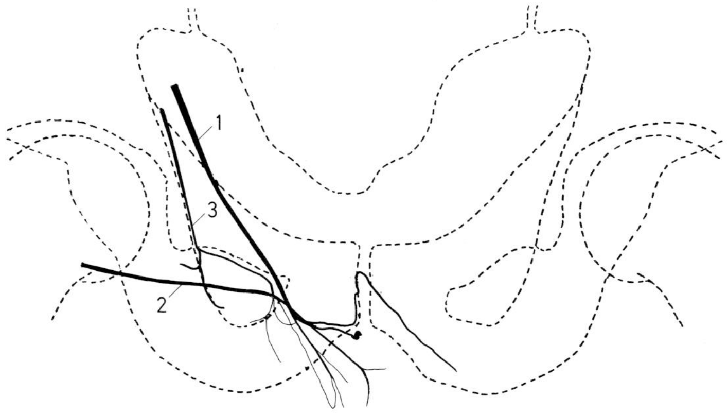

Fig. 75. Blood supply of the perineal region
1 internal pudendal artery
2 external pudendal artery
3 obturator artery

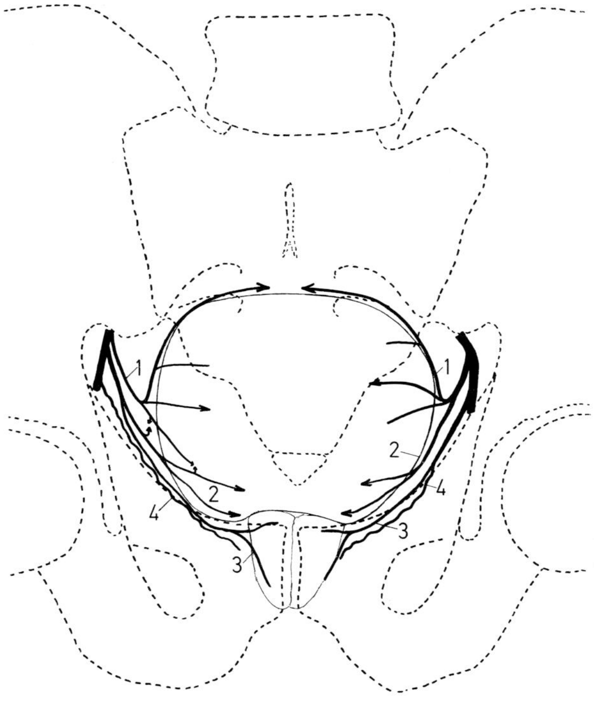

Fig. 76. Blood supply of the bladder
1 superior vesical artery
2 inferior vesical artery
3 prostatic artery
4 vesicular artery

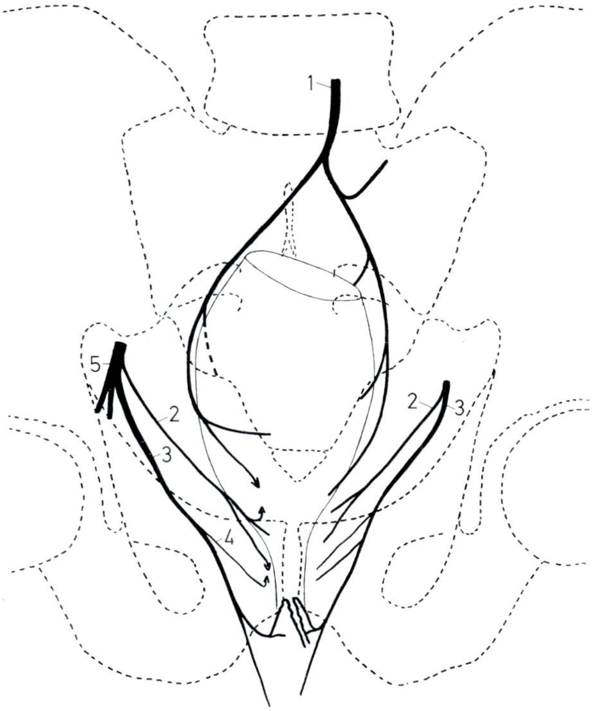

Fig. 77. Blood supply of the rectum
1 superior rectal artery
2 middle rectal artery
3 internal pudendal artery
4 inferior rectal artery
5 internal iliac artery

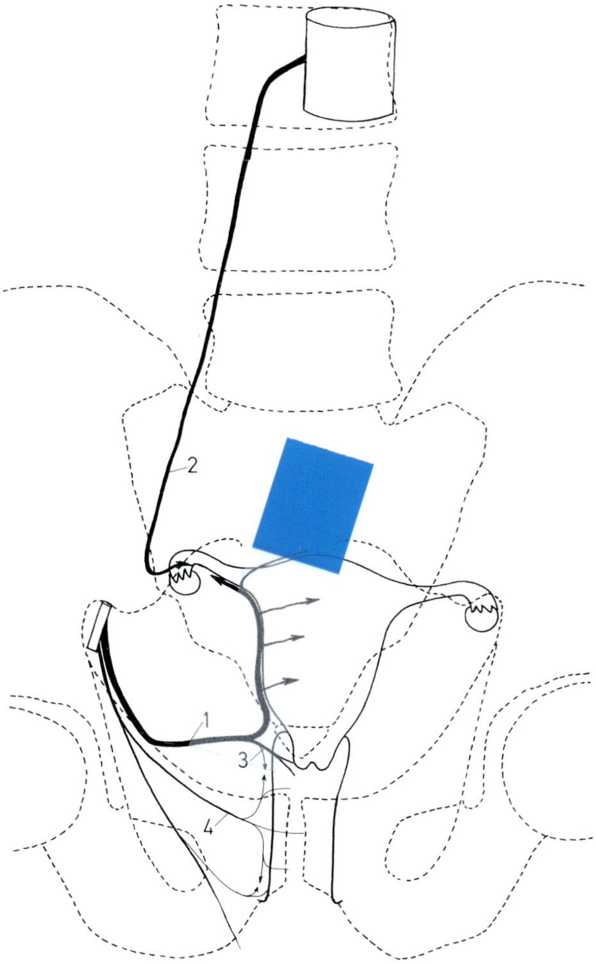

Fig. 78. Blood supply of the uterus
1 uterine artery
2 ovarian artery
3 cervicovaginal branch of the uterine artery
4 vaginal artery

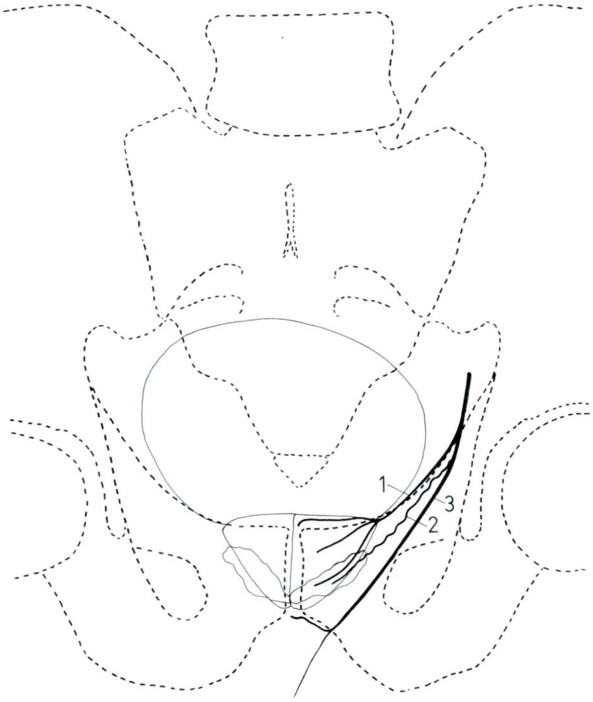

◁ **Fig. 79.** Blood supply of the accessory genital organs in the male
1 prostatic artery
2 vesicular artery
3 internal pudendal artery

4 Pathology

A. Introduction

The diagnosis of pelvic afflictions, excluding those which are purely vascular, is based upon clinical signs and, according to the situation, radiographic studies, endoscopy, ultrasounds, and CT scans. Today, resorting to arteriography is usually unnecessary. Nevertheless, arteriography is rightfully indicated in certain diagnostic situations (Lang 1970), particularly in preoperative evaluations, and it has new and major usefulness in therapeutic applications. These therapeutic applications include selective embolization, arterial dilatation, and, in the near future, selective injection of therapeutic agents.

B. Vascular Diseases

I. Arteritis

In cases of iliofemoral arteritis due to arteriosclerosis, aortic arteriography alone is adequate for the evaluation of the lesions (Fig. 80). Selective hypogastric arteriography is not indicated because collateral pathways make possible an appreciation of the state of the arterial axis situated downstream from an iliofemoral obstruction. Selective arteriography of branches of the hypogastric artery is indicated, however, in cases of inflammatory, infectious, and metabolic afflictions and aneurysms as well as other disturbances which may be responsible for erectile dysfunction (Lindenbaum et al. 1978) (Fig. 81).

II. Traumatic Vascular Lesions

Arteriography is indicated in two different circumstances:

1. Immediately following the traumatic incident in order to identify the site of bleeding and to perform hemostatic embolization (Marty et al. 1974; Paster et al. 1974; Perlberger 1977; Ring et al. 1974; Schroeder et al. 1978).
2. At a later stage, to evaluate the vascular lesions (arterial occlusions and aneurysms (Fig. 82) or posttraumatic A.V. fistula)

III. Vascular Malformations

Vascular malformations can be either congenital or acquired and can occupy the pelvic walls as well as the pelvic viscera. Before any therapeutic attempts, detailed arteriographic evaluation should be carried out in order to define their radioanatomic type (Neifeld et al. 1975; Olcott et al. 1976):

1. Simple arterial dysplasias which take the shape of aneurysms, stenoses, and multiple dilatations. They are encountered in certain cutaneomuscular arterial territories.
2. Direct arteriovenous fistulae are classically of traumatic origin; spontaneous types have, however, also been reported. They are efficiently cured by a detachable balloon or a coil.
3. Rapid blood flow arteriovenous malformations: they are defined arteriographically by dilated arteries, a more or less well-developed angiomatous network which is difficult to visualize because of the fast flow, and dilated, rapidly filled veins (Figs. 83, 84).

Only superselective arteriography enables a precise evaluation of these complex malformations by differentiating the various pedicles and individual angiomatous territories. Superselective arteriography is an indispensable first step toward therapeutic embolization. Today, embolization has completely transformed the prognosis of the se malformations by reducing the diversion of the blood flow and its consequences (functional, trophic, and hemorrhagic) and by reducing any eventual global hemodynamic repercussions. It can be used alone or as an ideal preoperative procedure in cases where excision is indicated, in order to avoid local recurrence. The advent of preoperative embolization followed by surgery has opened new avenues in the treatment of malformations previously considered inoperable.

The material used for embolization varies with the nature of the procedure; in preoperative procedures, Gelfoam; in therapeutic procedures, solid nonreabsorbable or liquid polymerizing agents. It should be noted that in these cases as well as others, arterial ligation performed at such a distance that arteriovenous shunts are not occluded presents certain risks, e.g., development of collateral pathways, and sometimes a sudden spurt in growth (Fig. 85). It should also be noted that our present knowledge cannot enable us to predict the evolution of these malformations. Therefore, a reasonable approach would be not to treat certain quiescent malformations which are discovered fortuitously.

IV. Capillary Vascular Malformations

Capillary, vascular malformations are predominantly represented by telangiectases and occasionally capillary hemangiomas. They are characterized by slightly dilated arterioles, a homogeneous pseudotumoral injection, and a poorly defined venous drainage. Embolisation is a very useful treatment, isolated or preoperative.

V. Capillary-Venular Vascular Malformations

Clinically such malformations are nonpulsating masses which become turgescent during effort and under increased venous pressure (Figs. 86, 87). They are characterized by normal feeding arterioles without arterial diversion, a slow progressive grapelike injection, and a lasting, stagnating, venous drainage. As a rule, only superselective arteriography may identify exactly these characteristics (Fig. 86). They are usually found associated with anomalies of larger venous vessels. Embolization can be used as either a preoperative or therapeutic measure.

VI. Venous Vascular Malformations

Venous vascular malformations usually concern the large venous trunks and can be associated with deep hypoplastic or normal veins. As a rule, these malformations are found associated with the previously cited malformations.

All of the aforementioned vascular malformations, regardless of their radioanatomic type, can be parietal (intra- or extrapelvic), visceral (vesical, genital, or rectal, Fig. 88), or mixed. Moreover, these malformations can be part of complex angiodysplastic syndromes: pelvic extension of an angioma of the lower extremity (Klippel-Trenaunay syndrome, Fig. 89); disseminated angiomas (Osler-Weber-Rendu or Bean's syndromes); cutaneous, visceral, bony, meningeal, or medullary metameric angiomas (Cobb's syndrome) which associate a pelvic angioma or an angioma of one of the extremities with a medullary angioma situated on that same metameric level (Fig. 90) (Djindjian).

Furthermore, the hypogastric artery is either the sole or the predominant afferent vessel in cases of vertebral angiomas, vertebromeningeal angiomas (Fig. 91), and meningeal, medullary, or meningomedullary angiomas (Fig. 92) (Heindel et al. 1975).

C. Tumoral Processes

Three different types of tumoral process can be defined according to their localization: parietal, neuronal, and visceral.

I. Parietal Tumors (Figs. 93, 94)

Arteriography is an excellent exploratory tool in the highly vascular parietal tumors; muscular, mesenchymatous tumors, lymph node sarcomas and especially primary or secondary bone tumors (renal, thyroid and mammary metastases) benefit from this technique. Although arteriography cannot usually indicate the benign or malignant nature of a neoplasm, it can accurately determine its degree of vascularization and the origins of its blood supply (WENGER et al. 1977). This makes possible an eventual preoperative or therapeutic embolization. Today, embolization has widened surgical solutions and modified the isotopic treatment of secondary bone sites of thyroid cancers.

II. Neuronal Tumors

Neuronal tumors, benign or malignant schwannomas, are rarely encountered. Selective arteriography reveals a mass which is supplied by the intrapelvic parietal branches of the hypogastric artery in most cases or less commonly by the lumbar or middle sacral arteries (Figs. 95, 96).
Embolization can facilitate surgical excision of these tumors, which tend to bleed profusely.

III. Visceral Tumors

Arteriography is rarely used in diagnosing visceral tumors (WINTERBERGER and MURPHY 1974; LANG 1967; GOERTTLER 1977), since clinical signs, radiographic studies, endoscopy, ultrasound, and CT scans are adequate. However, highly vascularized or highly hemorrhagic visceral tumors which necessitate palliative embolization are encountered because of their inoperative nature (MERLAND et al. 1974) (Figs. 97, 98, 101).

D. Hemorrhagic Syndromes

Selective pelvic arteriography is perhaps best suited for these disturbances. In bleeding due to trauma, arteriography makes possible precise localization of injury, and if indicated, hemostasis can be achieved by embolization. Vesical hemorrhages account for the greatest number of its applications:

1. In cases of hematuria due to cancer of the bladder (HIGGINS et al. 1977), superselective arteriography demonstrates a moderate degree of hypervascularization, giving a tumoral blush which is well visualized using a substraction technique (Fig. 19). Following irradiation this aspect is very different (NYLANDER et al. 1978); the arteries appear rigid and there is no blush.
2. When postirradiation bleeding occurs, embolization is the only alternative apart from total cystectomy, the prognosis of which is poor under such circumstances (Fig. 99) (CHIRAS et al. 1980).
3. Hematuria due to angiomas of the bladder is only rarely encountered.

I. Prostatic Hemorrhages

Prostatic hemorrhages can originate from tumoral processes (Fig. 101) or occur during prostatectomy (bleeding from the prostatic seat is increased by coagulation disturbances, e.g.; hemophilia, fibrinolysis). Embolization is remarkably effective in these cases (MITCHELL et al. 1976, MERLAND et al. 1974; PEREIRAS et al. 1977).

II. Rectal Hemorrhages

Carefully performed embolization of inoperable tumors and postirradiation bleeding is possible.

III. Genital Hemorrhages

The same applies to genital hemorrhages resulting from inoperable, recurring, or irradiated cervical or uterine sarcomas as to rectal hemorrhages. Arteriography, we will recall, is indicated in parametrial arteriovenous malformations (SCHWARZ et al. 1975; SMITH and WYATT 1977; BRAULT 1976) (Figs. 102–105).

E. Impotence

Arteriographic studies of the internal pudendal artery can reveal lesions responsible for erectile dysfunction (arterial thrombosis). They permit an evaluation for the possibility of corrective surgery.

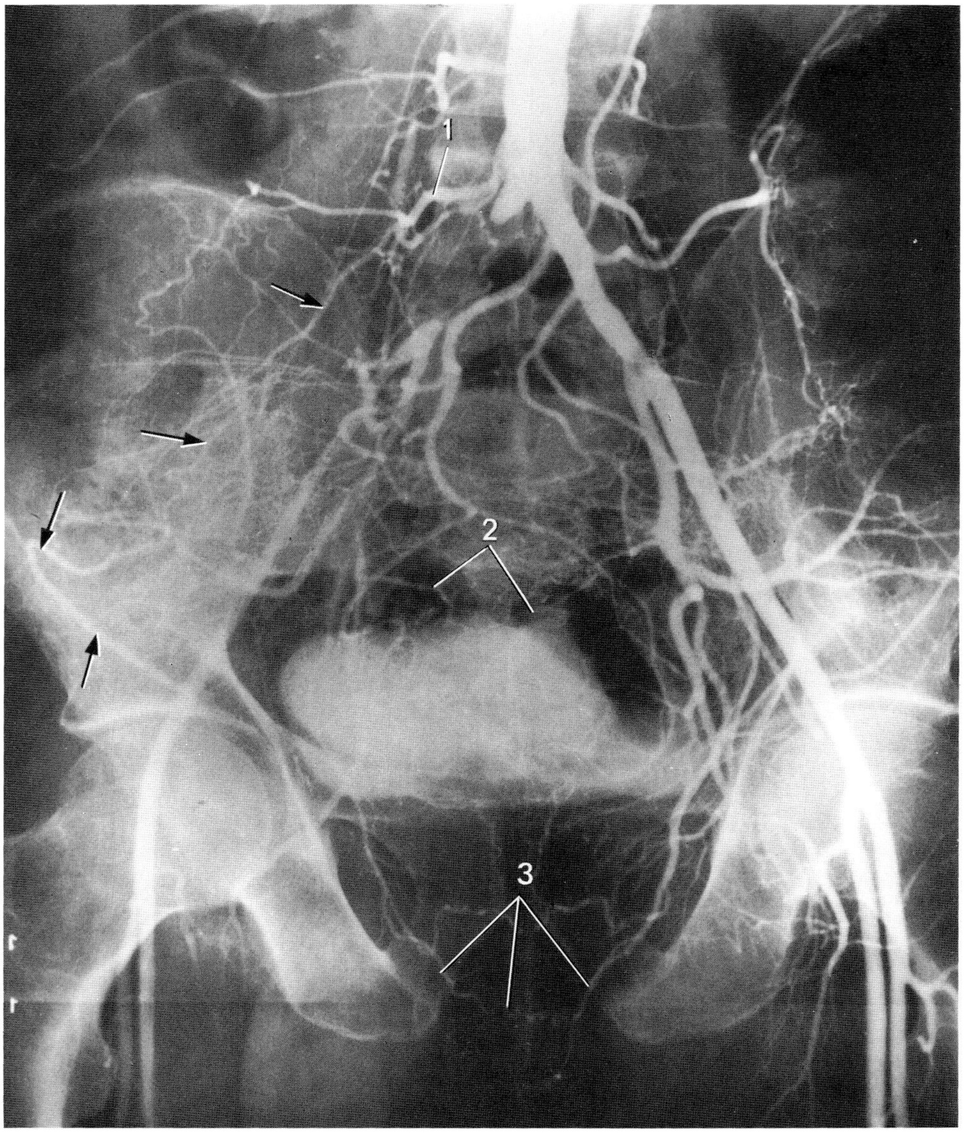

Fig. 80. Proximal occlusions of the common iliac artery and spontaneous recanalization of the femoral artery by anastomoses coming from the internal iliac artery and the deep circumflex iliac arteries. These anastomoses are longitudinal between the fourth lumbar and the deep circumflex iliac arteries; others are transversal [presacral (*2*) and perineal (*3*)] between the right and left internal iliac arteries

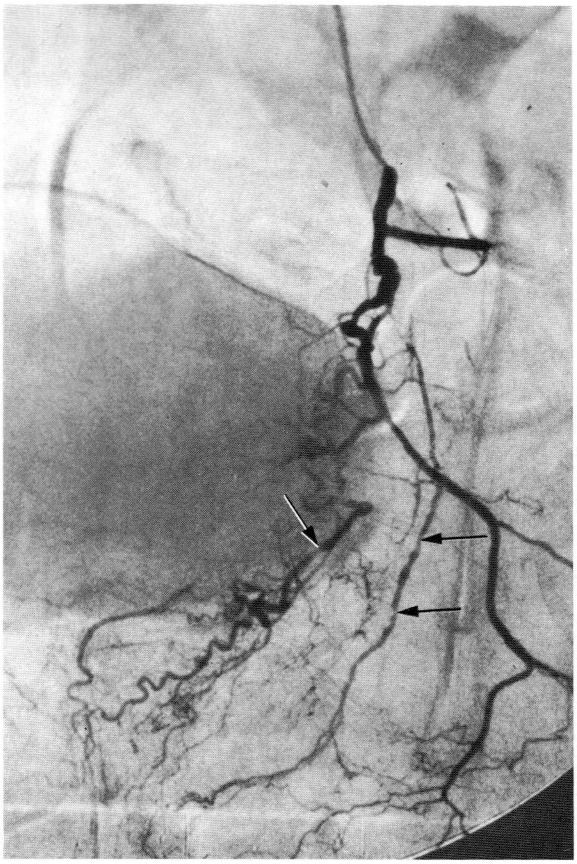

Fig. 81. Several stenoses on the trunk and the branches of the internal pudendal artery in a case of diabetes mellitus (*arrow*)

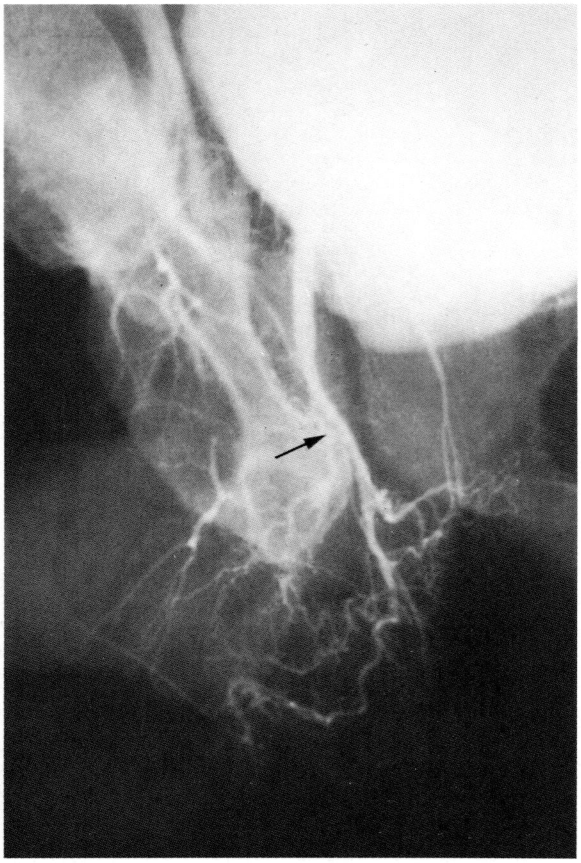

Fig. 82. Posttraumatic impotence: oblique view shows an aneurysm (*arrow*) on the perineal part of the internal pudendal artery with occlusion of the dorsal artery of penis

Fig. 83 a–e. Young woman suffering from pain and uterine bleeding. The clinical examination revealed a bruit. Angiography shows an arteriovenous fistula in the parametrium. It was successfully treated by embolization and surgical removal. **a** Aortography: on the left side, extremely rapid opacification of the veins (*1*), which present 2 large dilatations (*2*) separated by stenoses. On the right side, hypertrophic uterine artery with important transverse anastomoses (*3*). **b** Selective arteriography of the left uterine artery: several hypertrophied branches running into a very large internal iliac vein. The area of the arteriovenous shunting is very limited. **c** Left uterine artery after embolization. **d** Left internal iliac artery after embolization: complete occlusion of the feeding arteries of the fistula. **e** Right internal iliac artery: contralateral anastomoses via the branches of the right uterine artery supply the fistula but with a very slow flow ▷

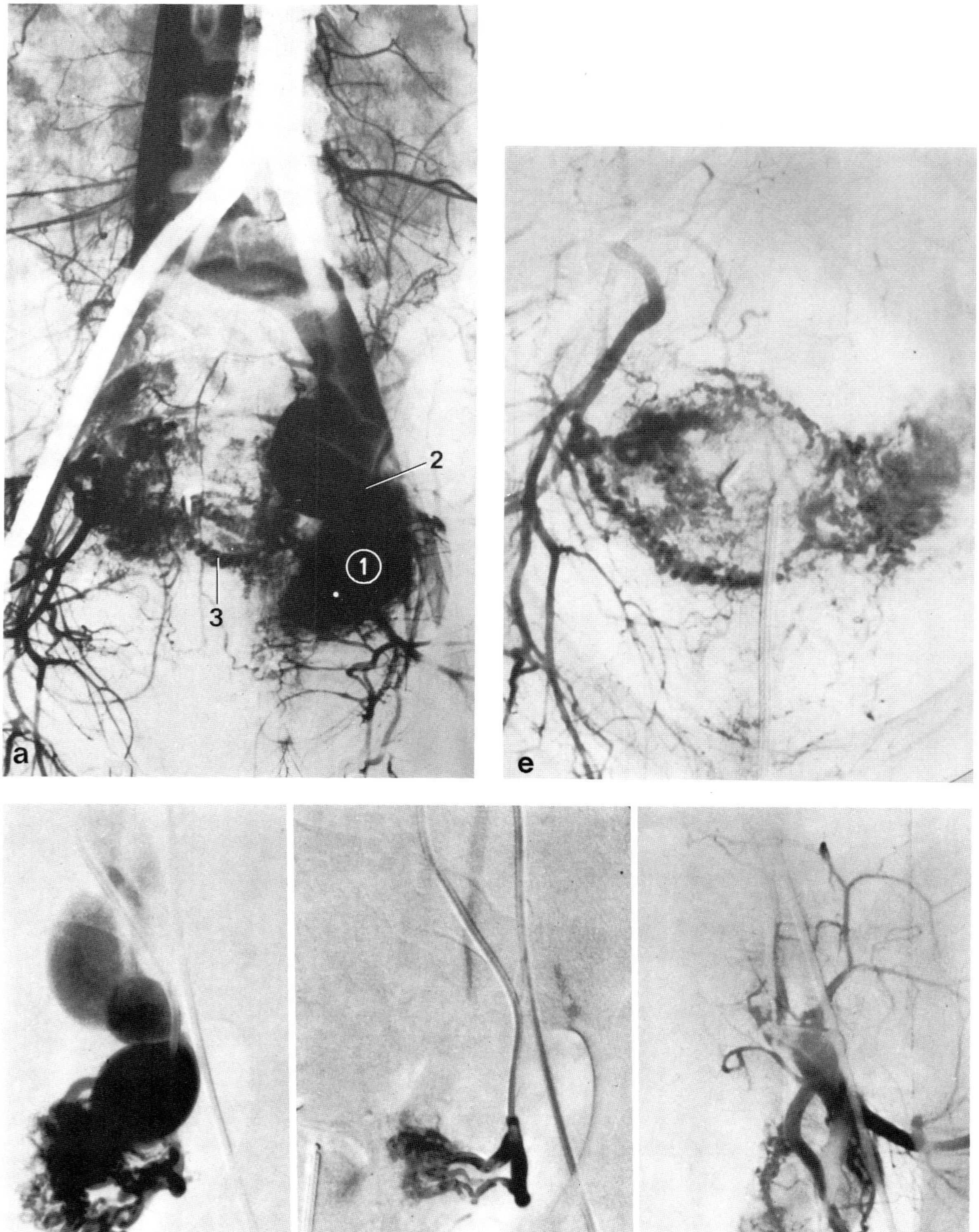
2
1
3
a
e
b
c
d

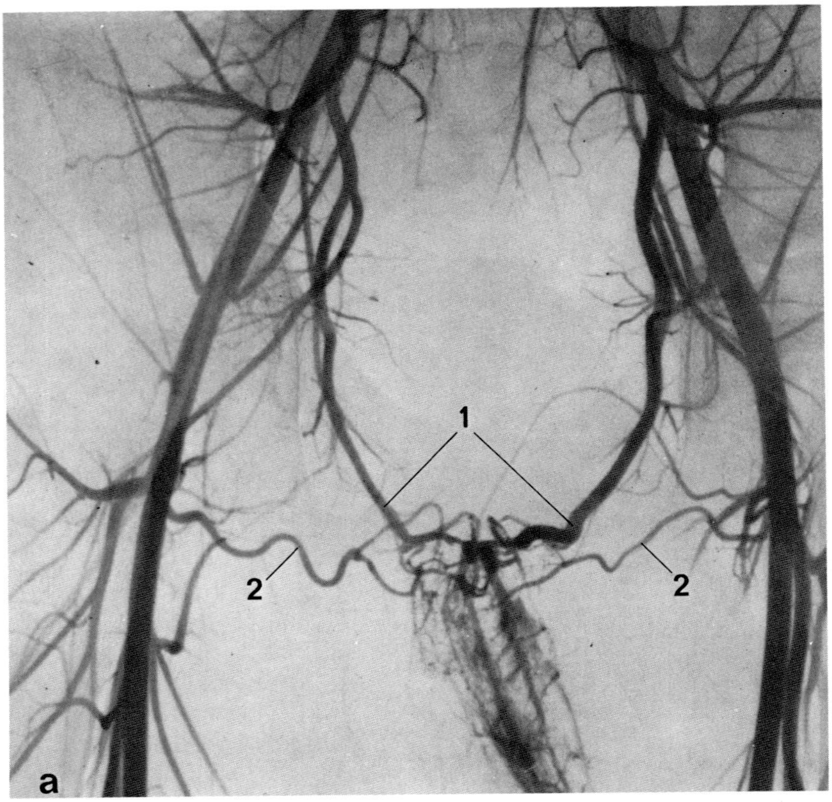

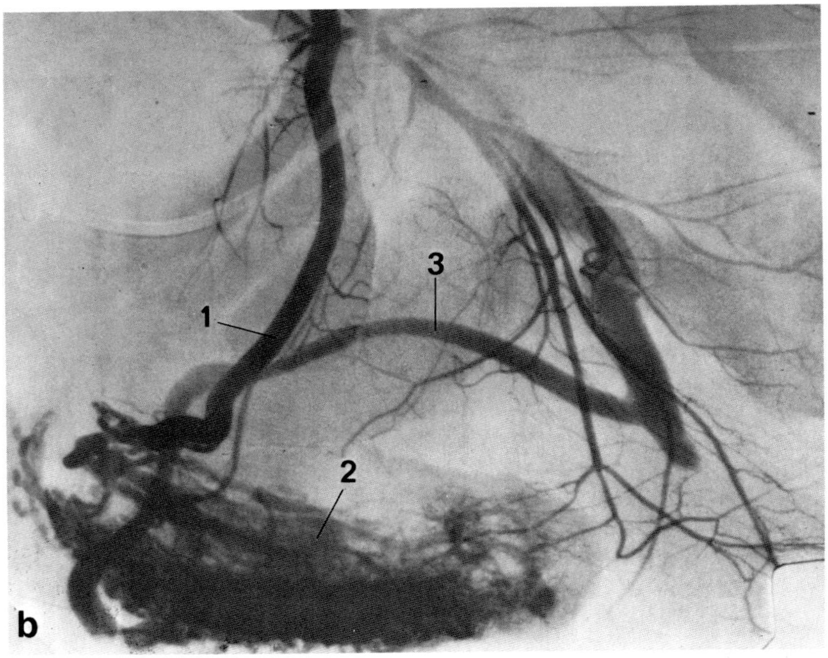

Fig. 84 a–f. Large arteriovenous angioma of the penis with hypertrophied arteries and an extremely rapid venous drainage. This patient suffers from priapism, bleeding and anemia. The embolization stabilized the angioma and permitted healing of the cutaneous lesions. **a** Aortography: the angioma is supplied by both internal (*1*) and external (*2*) pudendal arteries. **b** Left internal iliac artery: hypertrophic internal pudendal artery (*1*), dysplastic intermediate network (*2*) and rapid venous phase via the external pudendal vein (*3*).

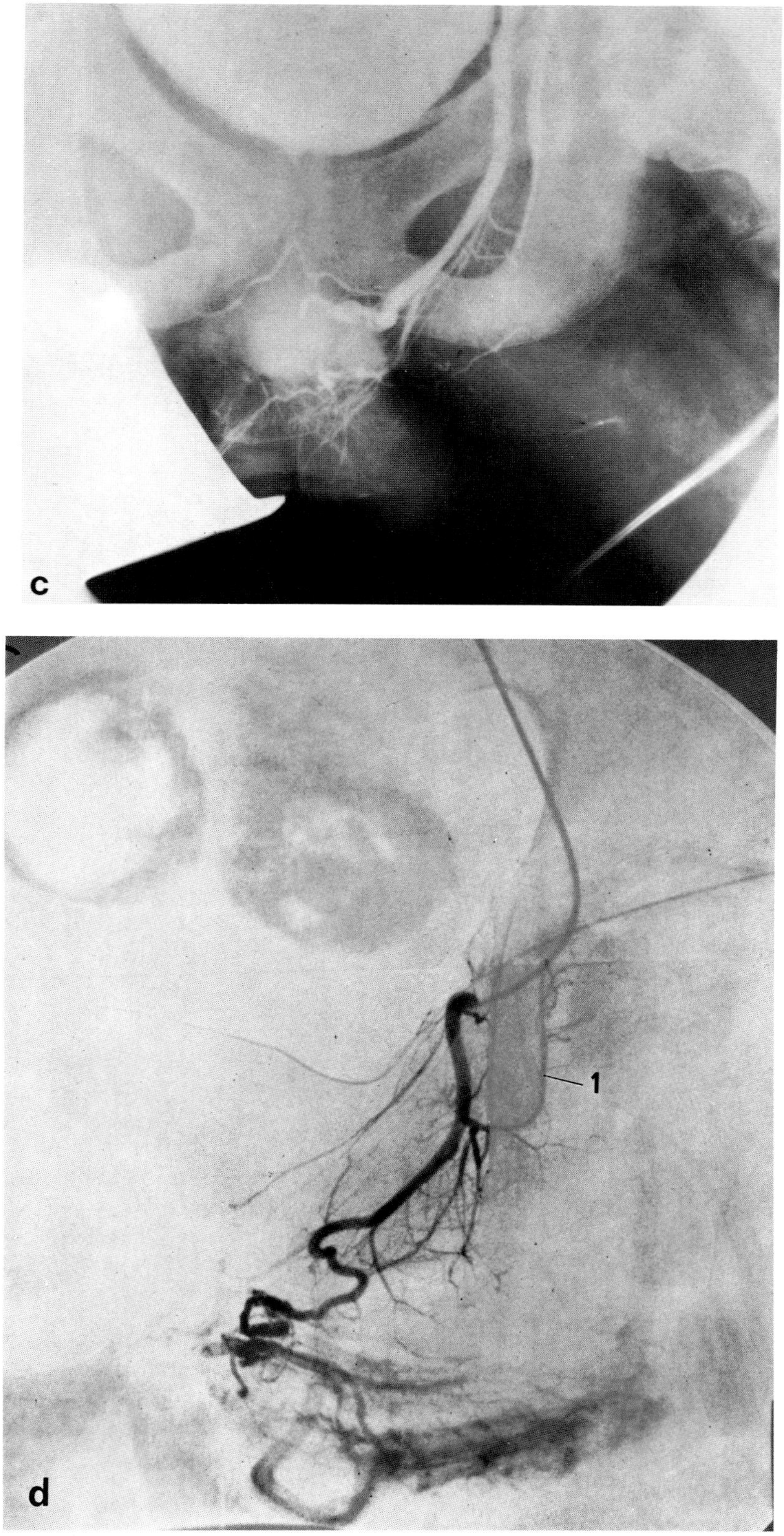

Fig. 84. c After embolization of the left internal pudendal artery the angiomatous network has disappeared. **d** The left obturator artery (which arises, from the external iliac artery) supplies the angioma; *1* acetabular branch

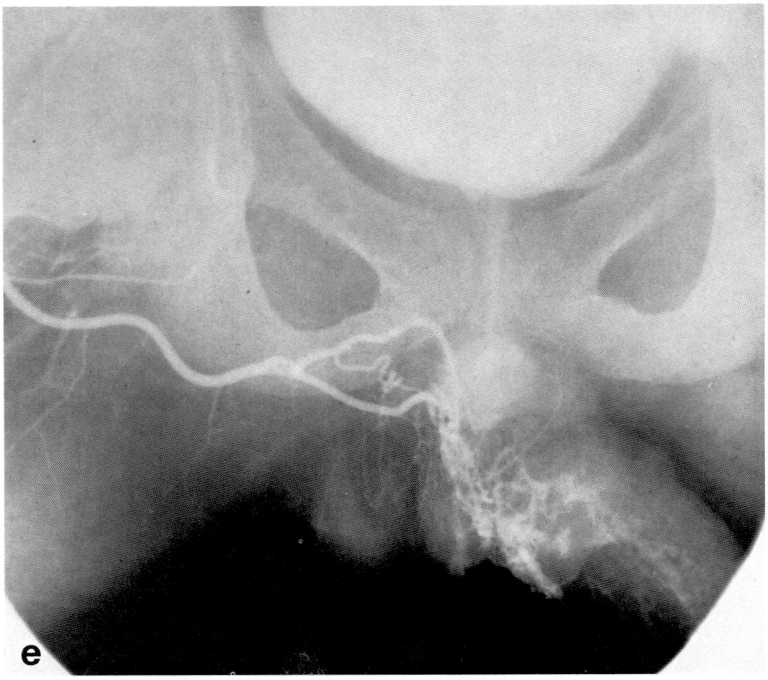

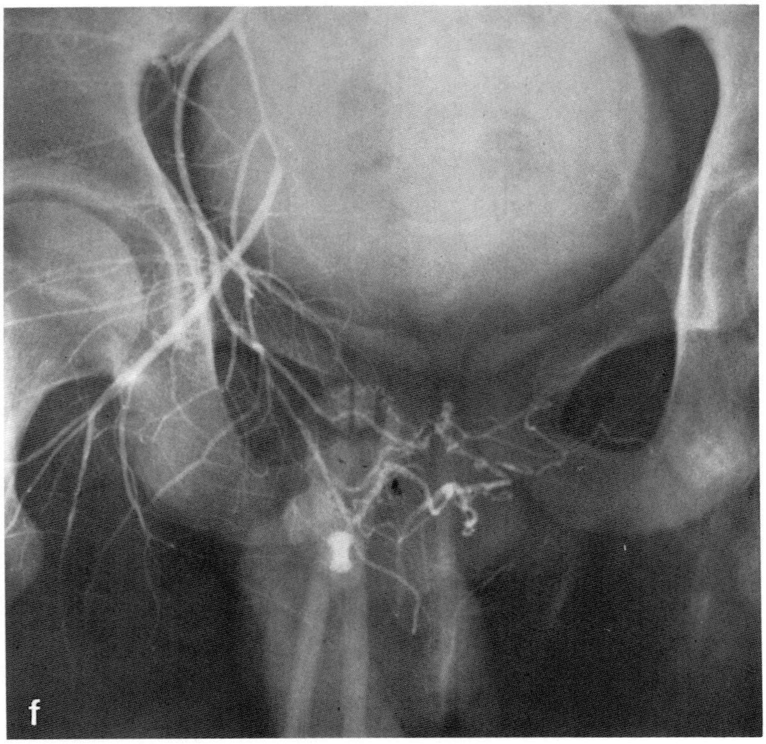

Fig. 84. e Supply from the right external pudendal artery. **f** Aortography after embolization of the various pedicles

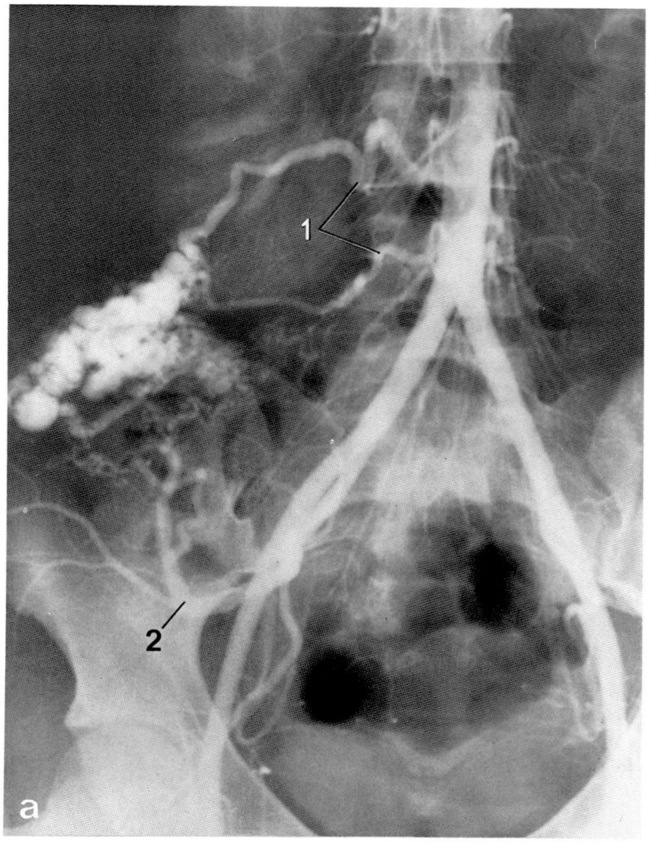

Fig. 85 a–h. 16 year-old-girl with a pulsating mass in the right gluteal region. **a** The aortography shows a voluminous arteriovenous angioma supplied by the third and fourth lumbar arteries (*1*) and the superficial branch of the superior gluteal artery (*2*). As it was not possible to remove the angioma surgically, ligation of the main pedicles was performed

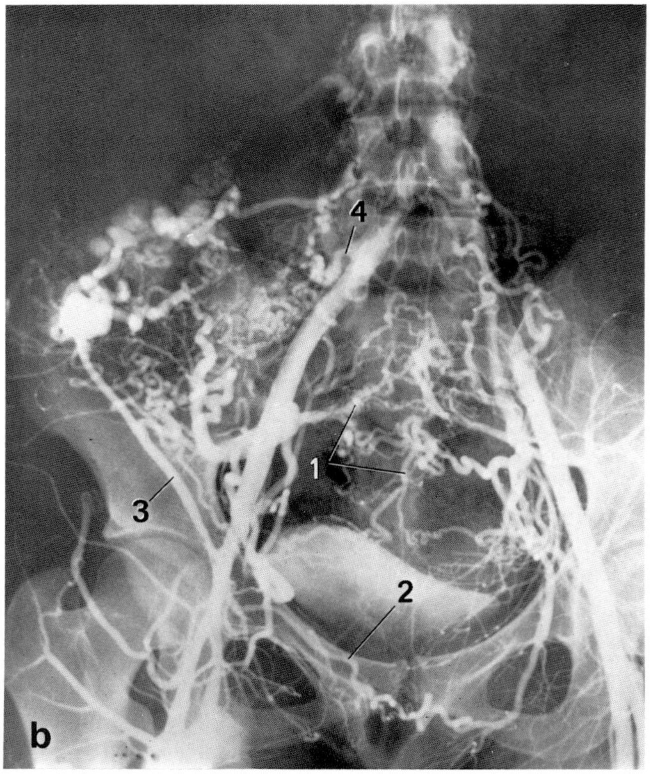

Fig. 85. b After ligation of the internal iliac and the third and fourth lumbar arteries, we can see the dilatation of many anastomoses: contralateral [presacral (*1*) pubic (*2*)] and iliac [deep circumflex iliac artery (*3*), fifth lumbar artery (*4*)]

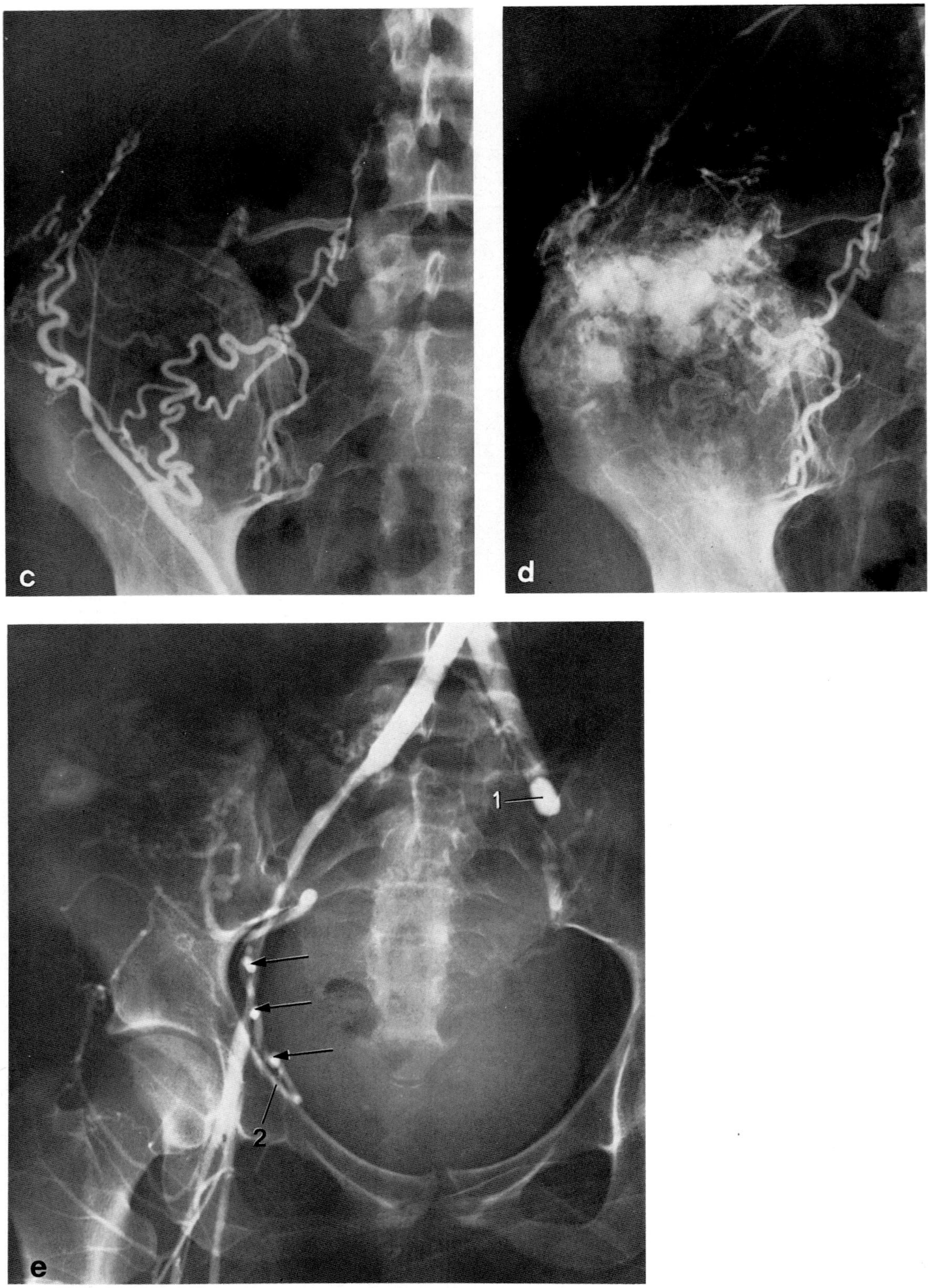

Fig. 85. c, d Deep circumflex artery supplying the malformation via anastomatic channels. **e** Temporary occlusion by a balloon catheter (*1*) of the opposite common iliac artery: it becomes evident that a direct connection exists between the inferior epigastric artery (*2*) and the vascular malformation via the retrograde filling of the obturator artery (*arrows*)

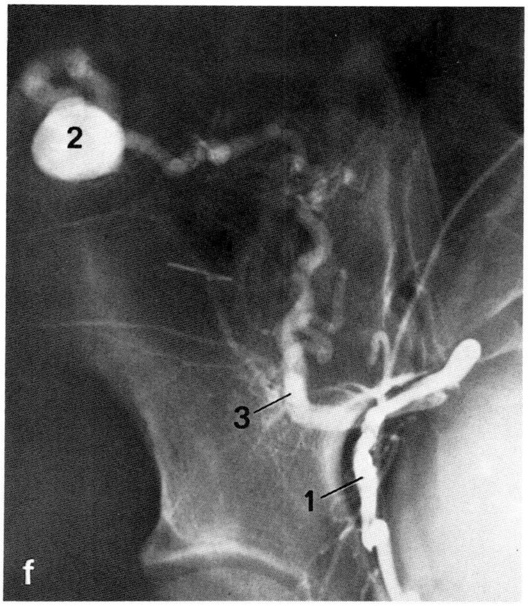

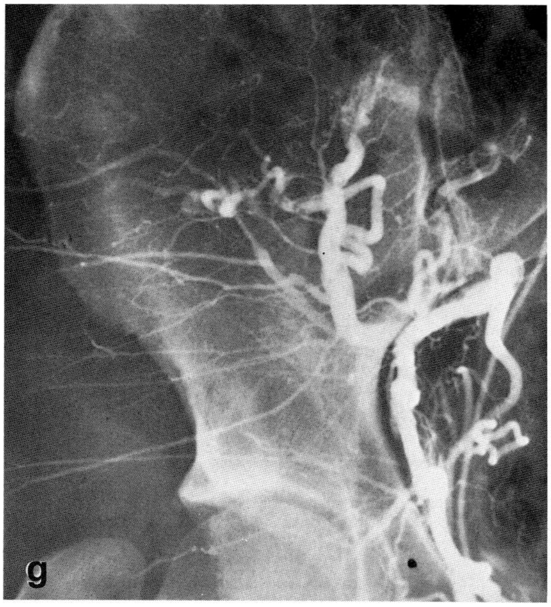

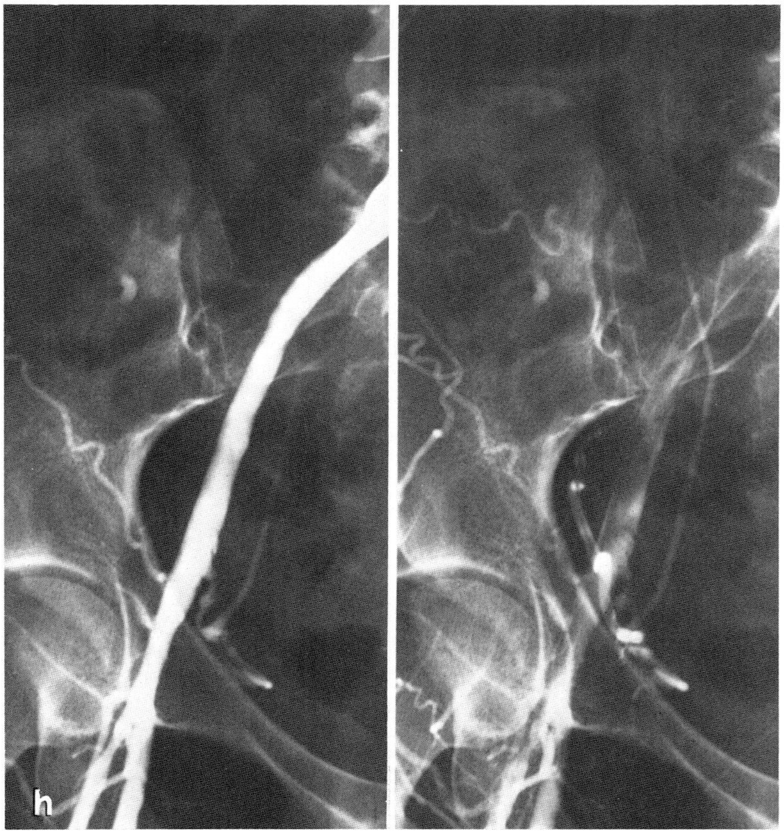

Fig. 85. f Hyperselective catheterization of the right inferior: the retrograde filling of the obturator artery (*1*) epigastric artery opacifies the angioma (*2*) via the superior pudendal artery (*3*). The embolization was performed under temporary balloon occlusion of the common iliac artery on the opposite side. **g** Control after embolization through the inferior epigastric artery: the malformation has disappeared. **h** Common iliac artery after embolization with disappearance of the arteriovenous malformation. This permitted the bloodless surgical removal of the entire angioma without functional damage

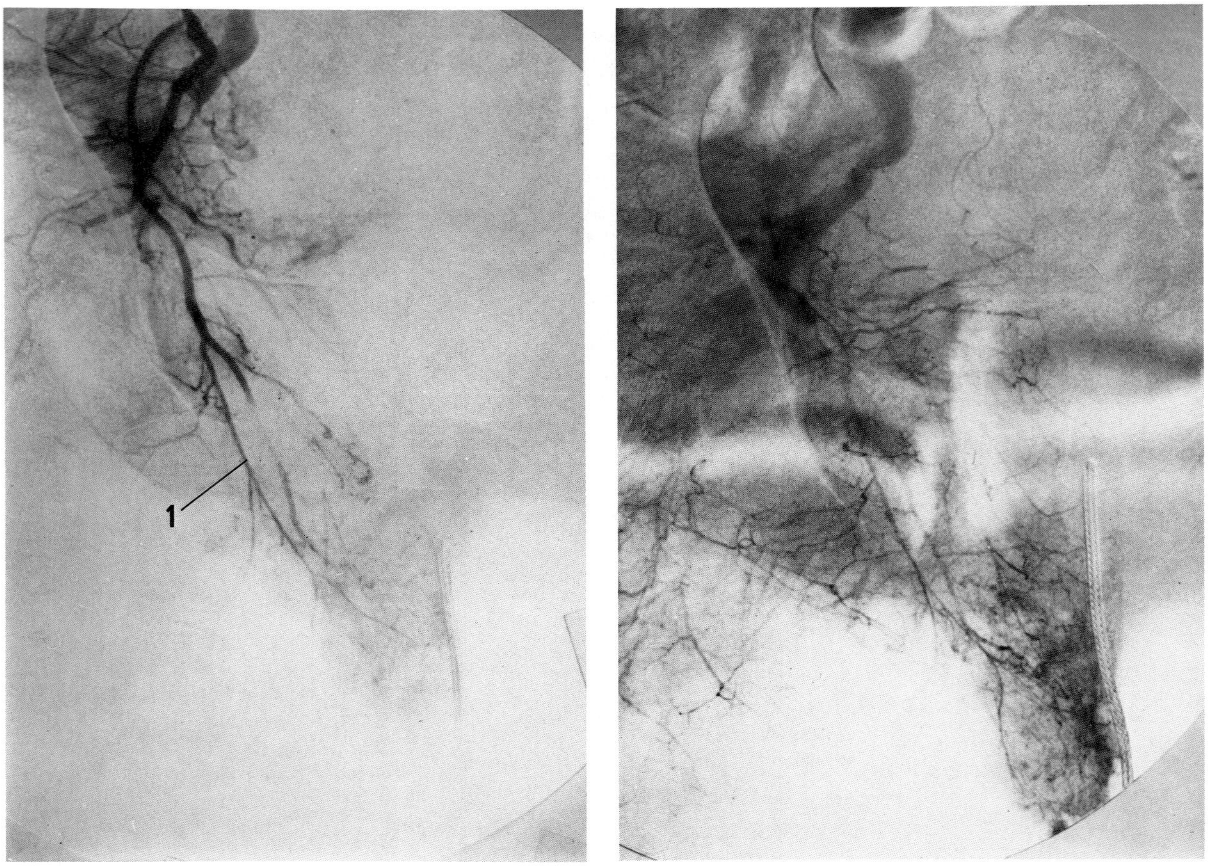

Fig. 86. Capillarovenous angioma of the right labium majus pudendi: superficial perineal artery (*1*) and the artery of the labium majus pudendi are normal but there is a blush on the capillary phase which persists on the later films

Fig. 87 a–f. Capillarovenous angioma of the labium majus pudendi in a case of Klippel-Trenaunay syndrome on the ipsilateral limb. **a** Internal pudendal artery: on the capillary phase venous lakes appear on the internal part of the limb. **b** Internal iliac artery: opacification of the venous lakes ▷

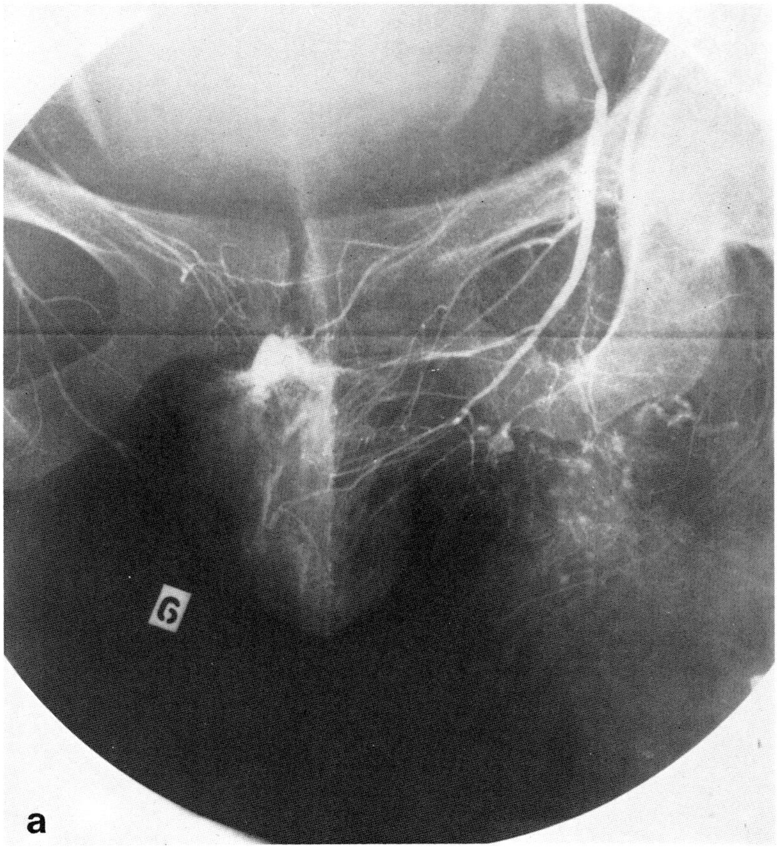

a

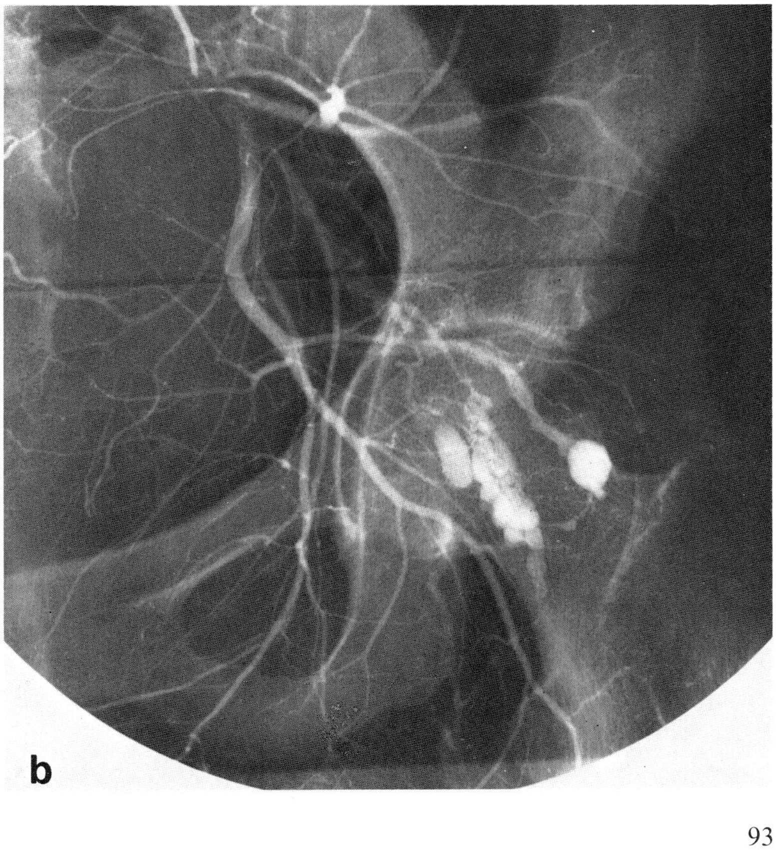

b

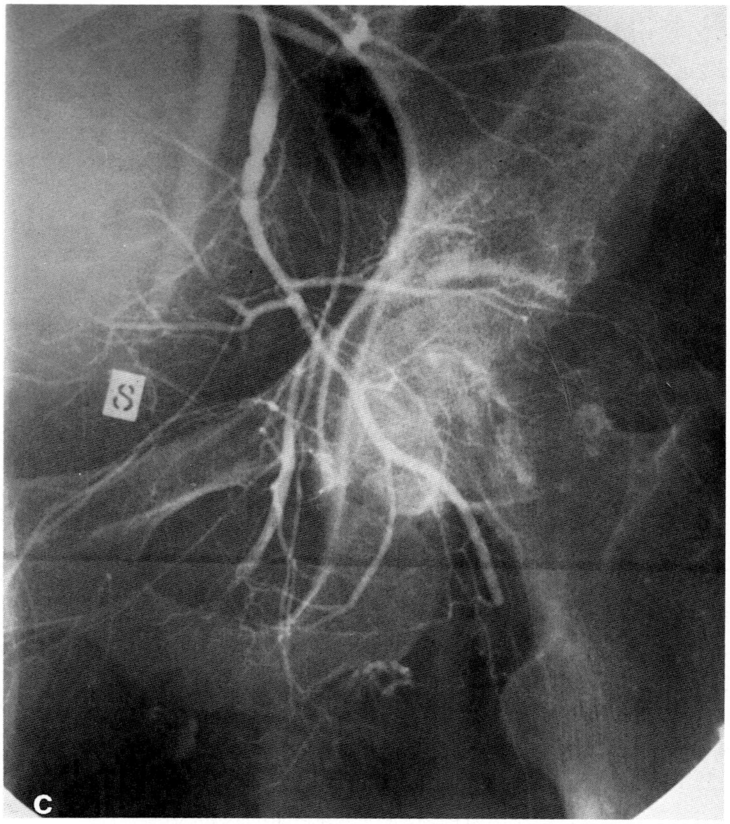

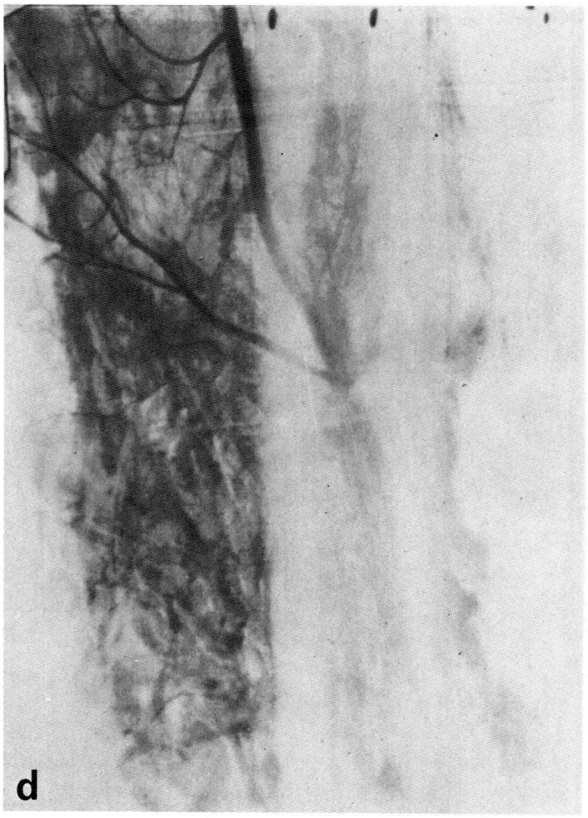

Fig. 87. c After embolization of the inferior gluteal artery the venous lakes disappear. **d** On the thigh there is a diffuse capillarovenous malformation

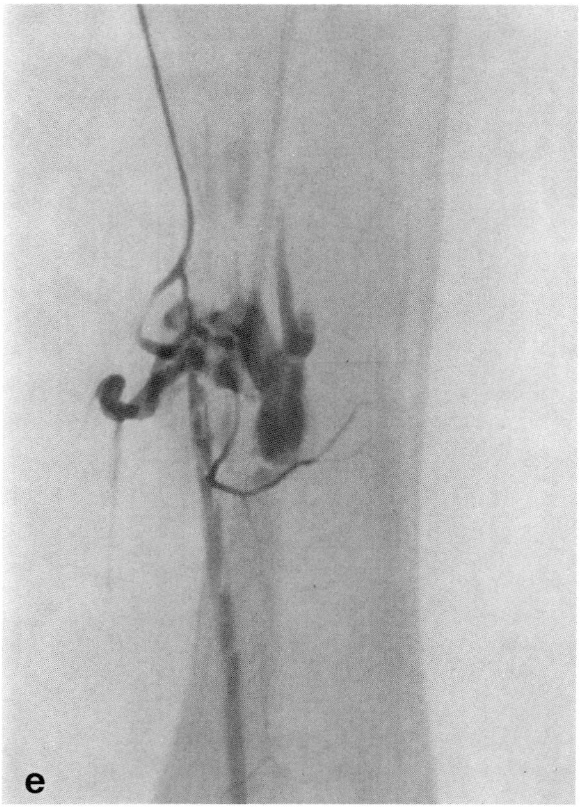

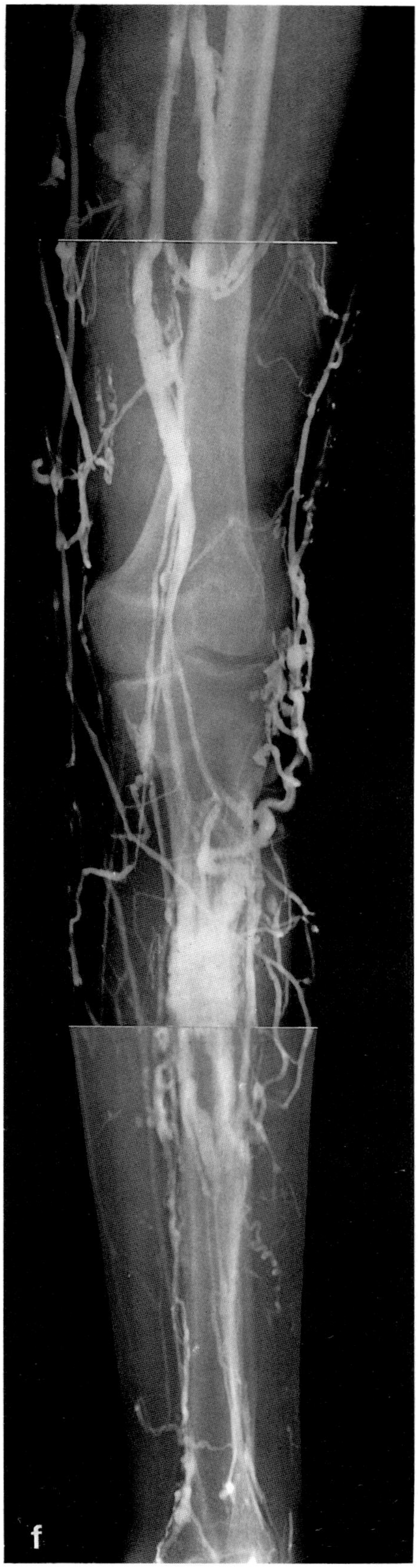

Fig. 87. e At the same level there are localized arteriovenous shunts. **f** Phlebography of the limb shows a diffuse venous dysplasia

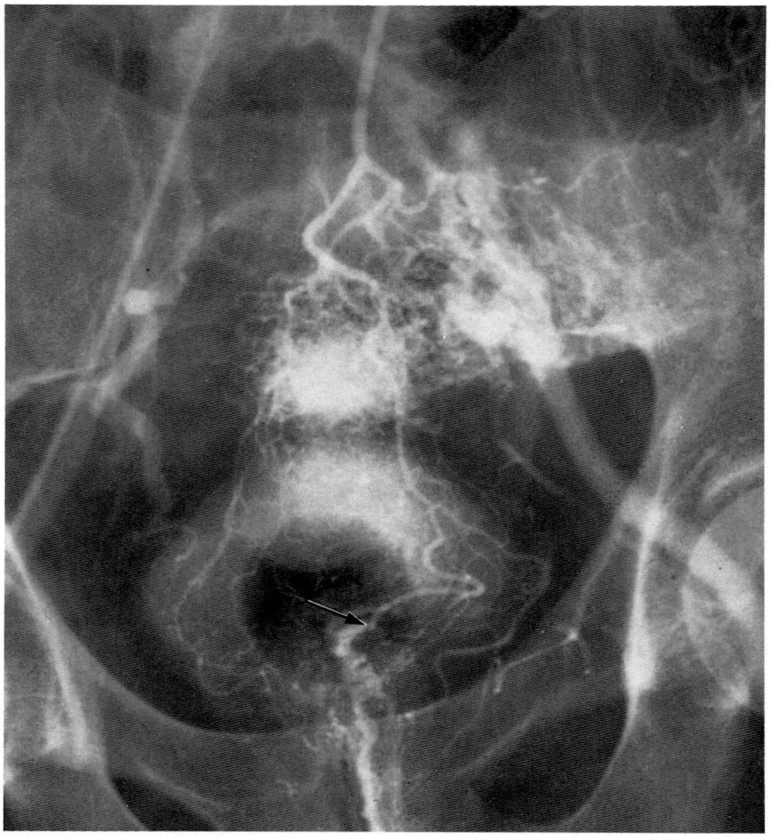

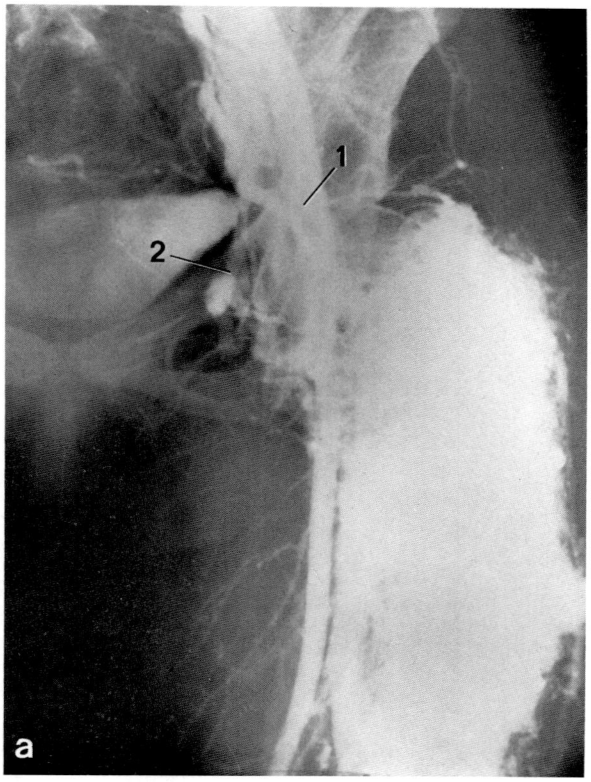

△
Fig. 88. Massive rectal bleeding with normal rectoscopy. Arteriography reveals an arteriovenous fistula of the anal canal (*arrow*)

Fig. 89 a–d. Arteriovenous angioma of the thigh in a 14-year-old girl who was surgically treated at the age of 18 months for a congenital dysplasia of the hip. At the time of investigation she presented isolated cardiac failure with a cardiac output at 12,71 mn. **a** Aortography: enormous angioma of the thigh supplied by branches of the deep and superficial femoral arteries the inferior gluteal artery (*1*) and the obturator (*2*) artery

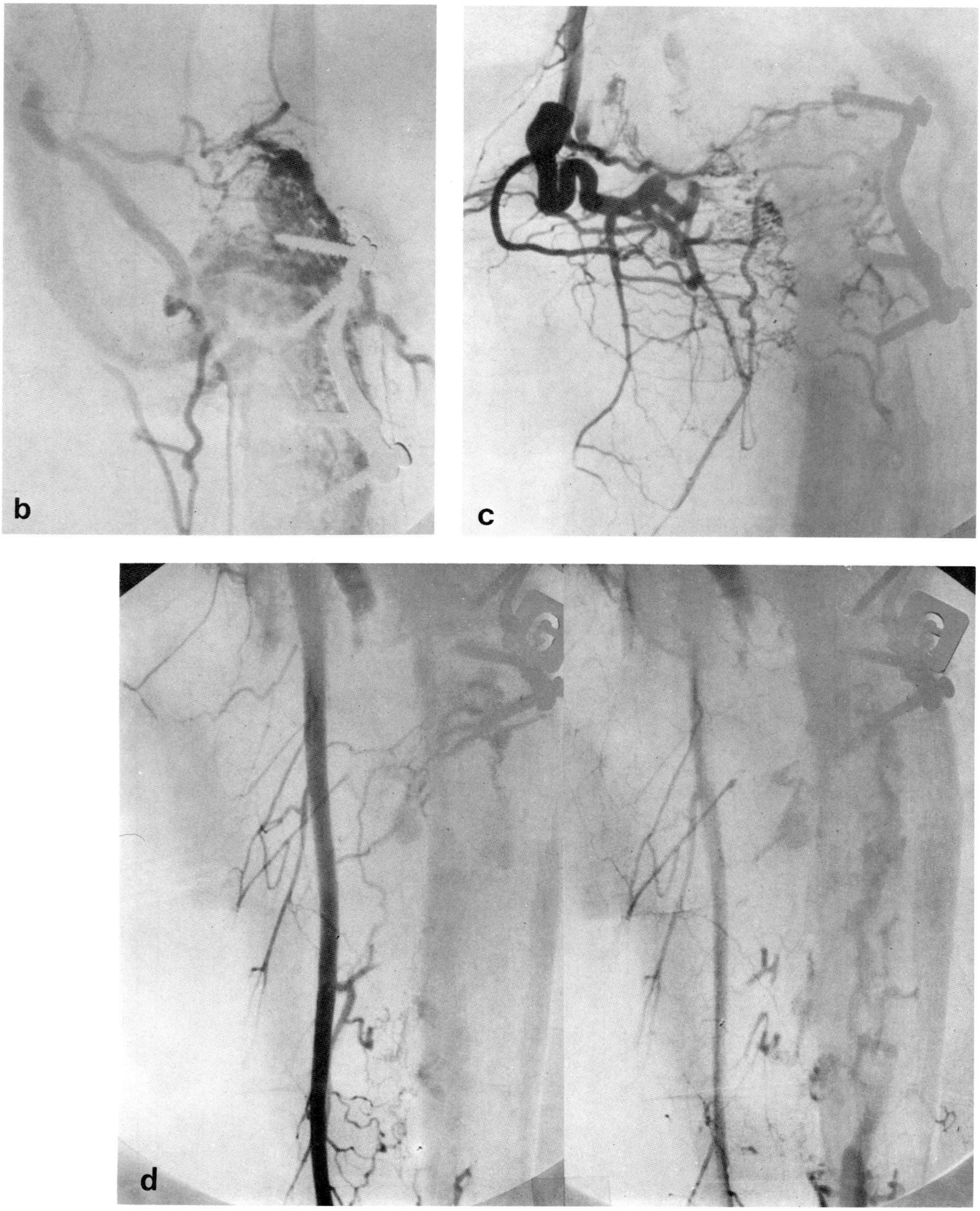

Fig. 89. b Inferior gluteal artery. **c** Obturator artery: dilatation of its external branch. **d** Six weeks after embolization (cardiac output 4,71)

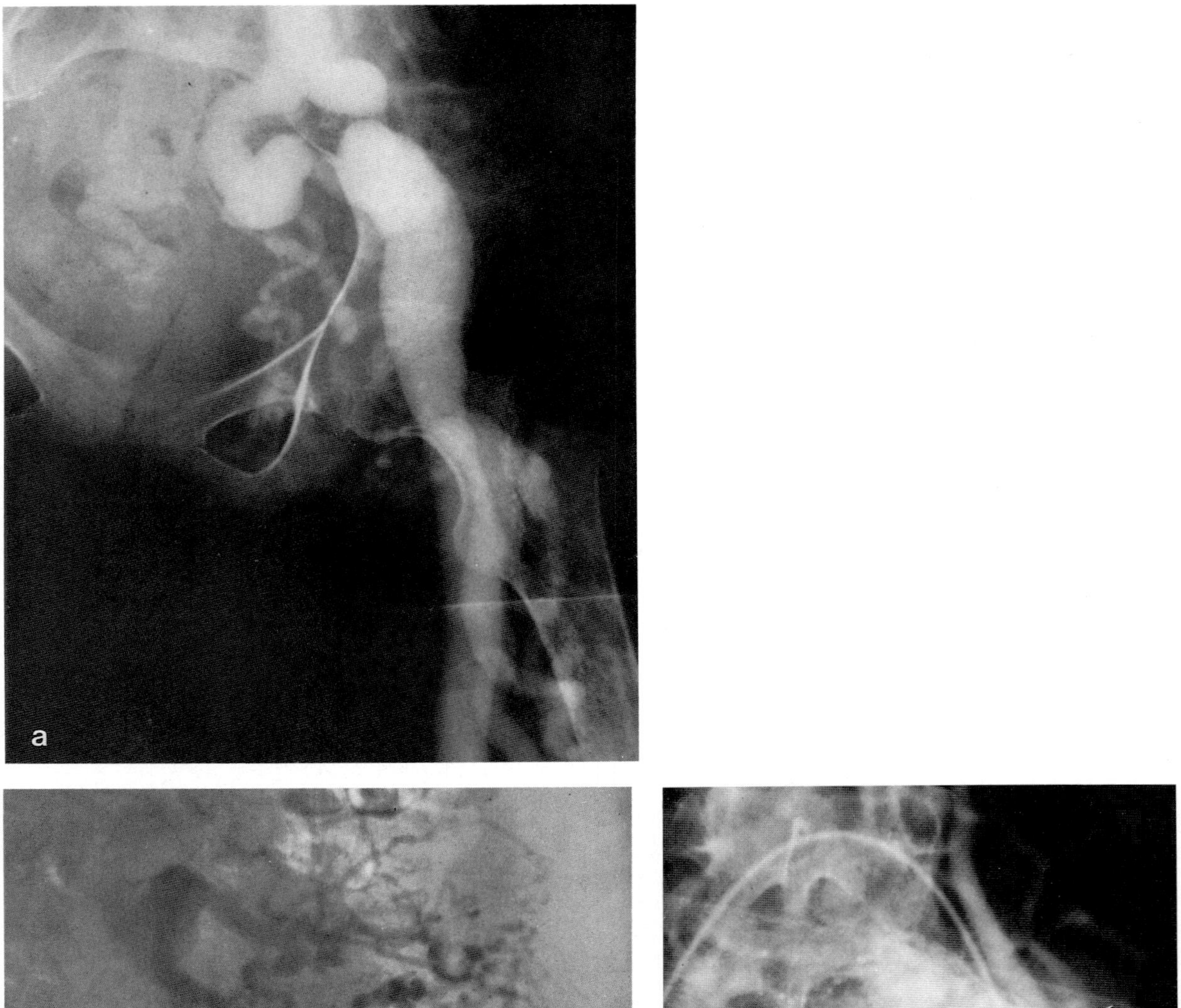
a
b
c

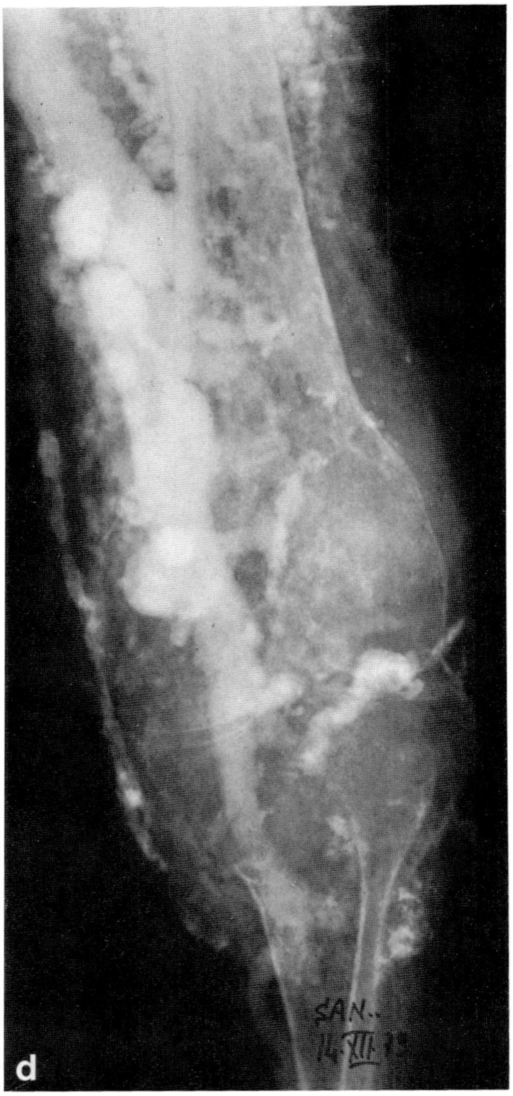

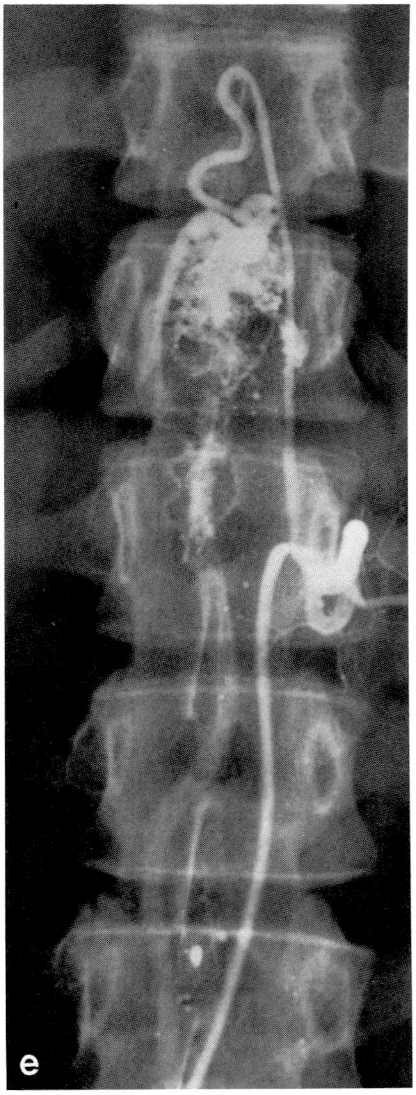

Fig. 90 a–e. Arteriovenous angioma (Klippel-Trenaunay-Weber) associated with a metameric vertebro-medullary angioma. **a, b** Aortography: dilatation of all the arteries of the limb with osseous modification secondary to the functional incapacity. **c** Internal iliac artery: hypertrophic iliolumbar artery (*arrow*) supplying the vertebral angioma (L-5). **d** Later phase. **e** Spinal angioma supplied by the artery of Adamkiewicz

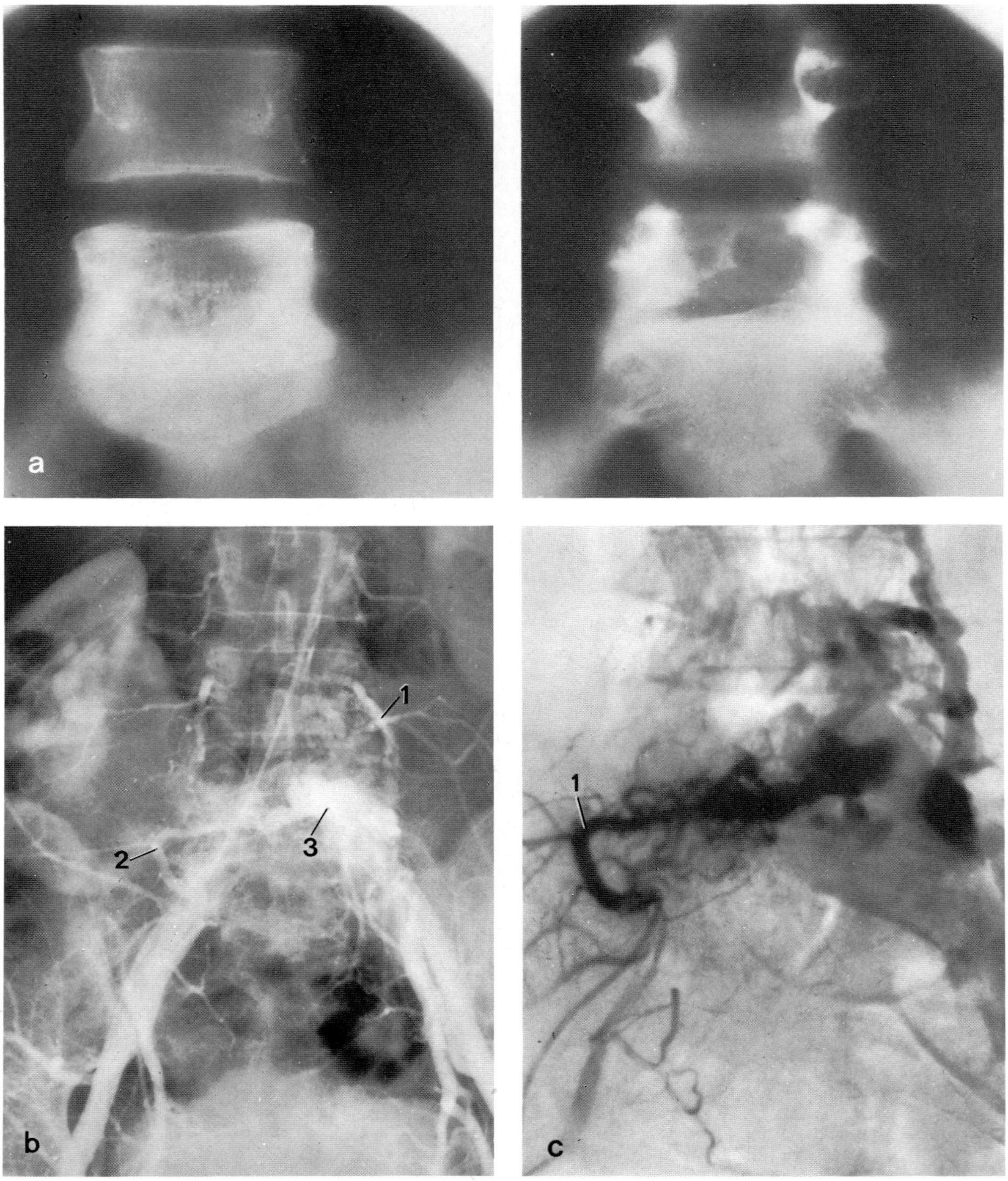

Fig. 91 a–c. Arteriovenous spinal angioma with associated dural arteriovenous fistula at the L-5 level, in a young women suffering from lumbar pain and sciatica. Normal radiculography. **a** Anterior tomography of the vertebral body shows a typical aspect of a vertebral angioma. On a more posterior section, there is a round lacuna which is due to a large epidural venous ectasia draining the fistula.

b Aortography: the fourth lumbar artery (*1*) and the right iliolumbar artery (*2*) feed the angioma (*3*).

c Right iliolumbar selective angiography (*1*). It opacifies the epidural fistula and the epidural venous ectasia, which is in close contact with the eroded bone as seen on tomography

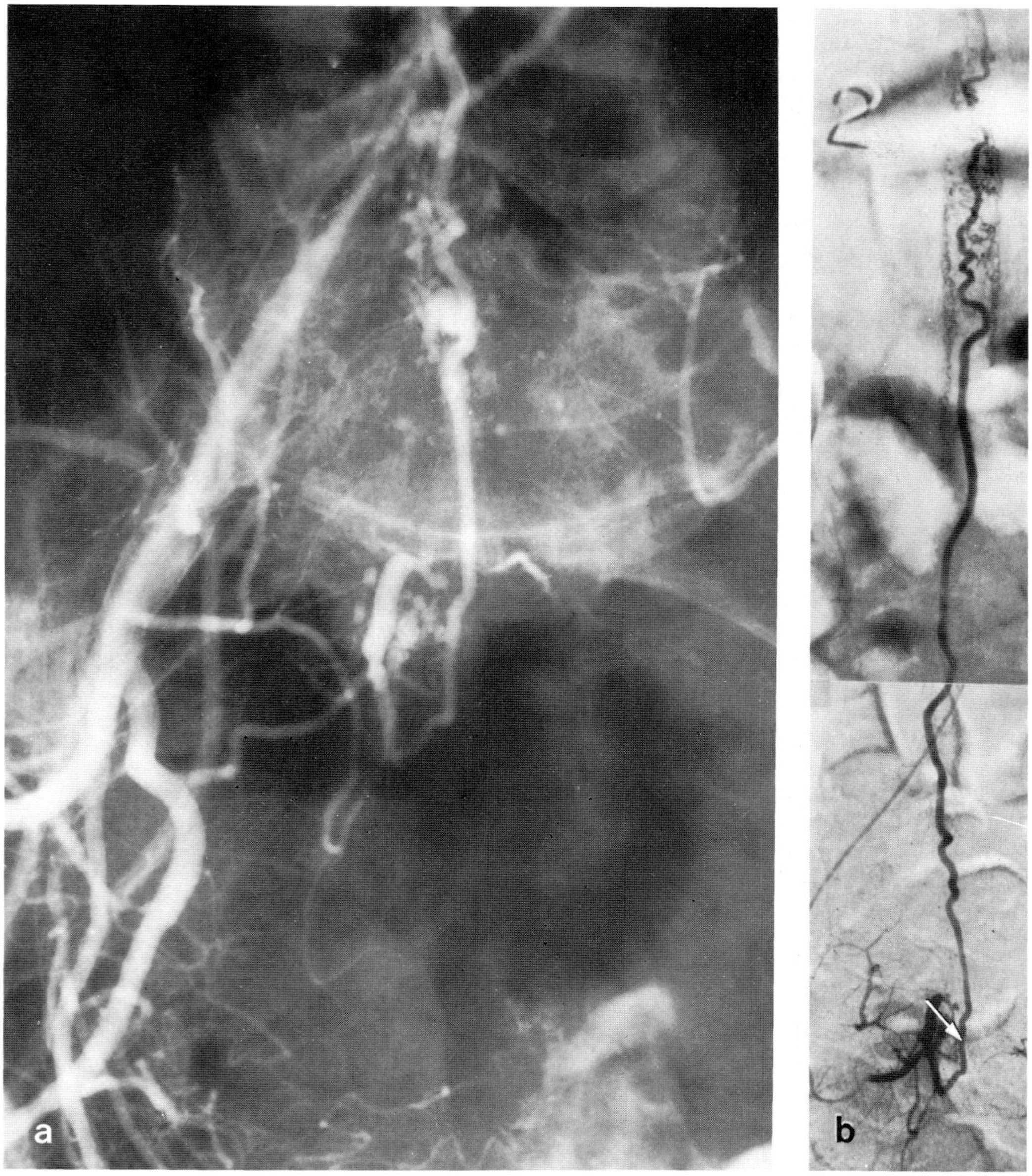

Fig. 92 a–e. Progressive paraplegia with vascular anomalies on the myelograph. Selective injection of the right internal iliac artery (**a**) shows an ascending opacification of an abnormal intradural vessel fed by the lateral sacral artery and by a proximal branch of the inferior gluteal artery. **b** Selective opacification of the branch of the inferior gluteal artery: it confirms the arteriovenous fistula (*arrow*) in front of the second sacral notch. On the lateral view

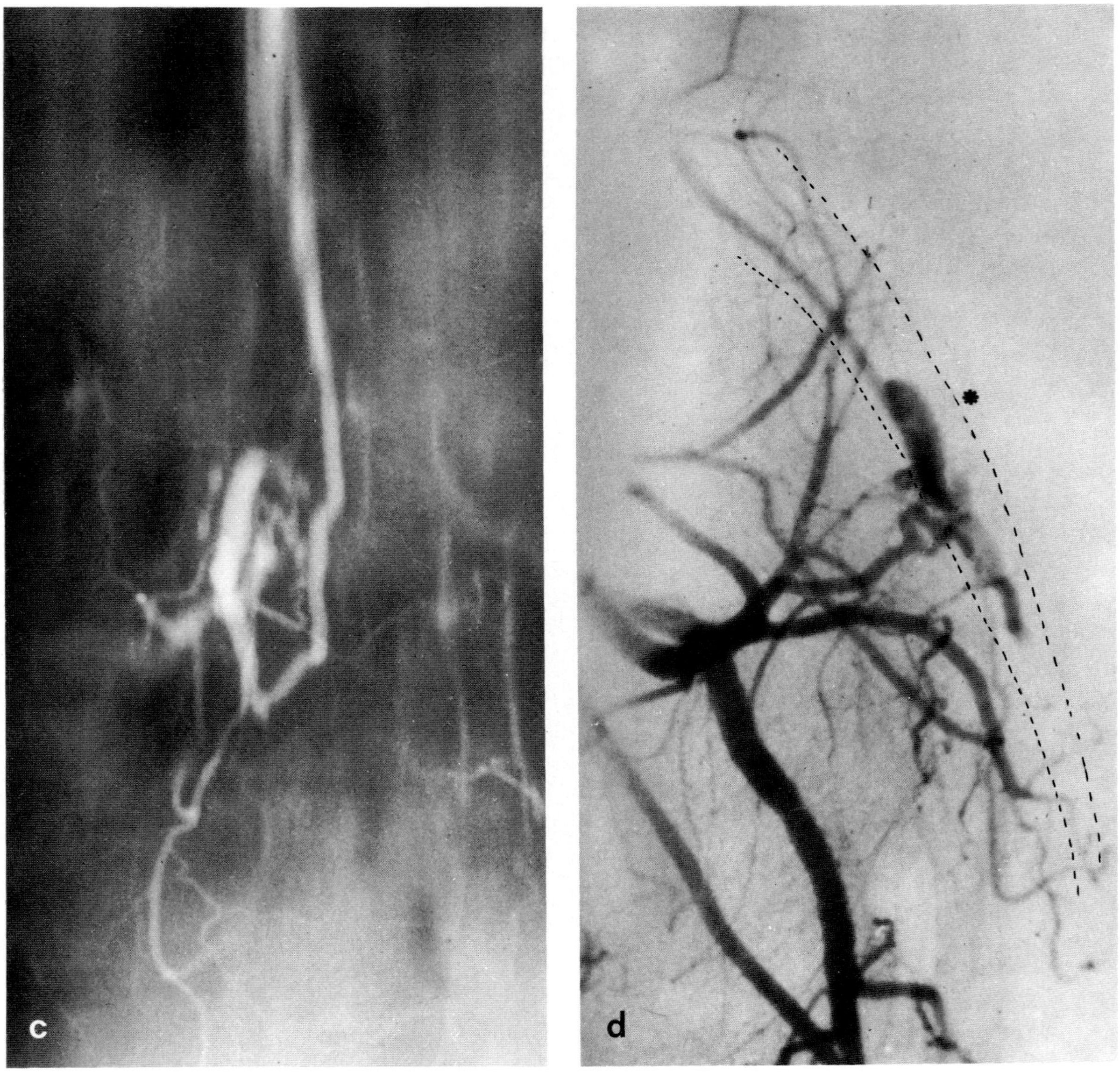

Fig. 92. c This fistula is on the anterior part of the sacral canal. With angiotomography **d** the fistula is better visualized. The ascending vein is the vein of the filum terminale. It drains into the dilated perimedullary veins, which are dilated up to the dorsal region (**b**)

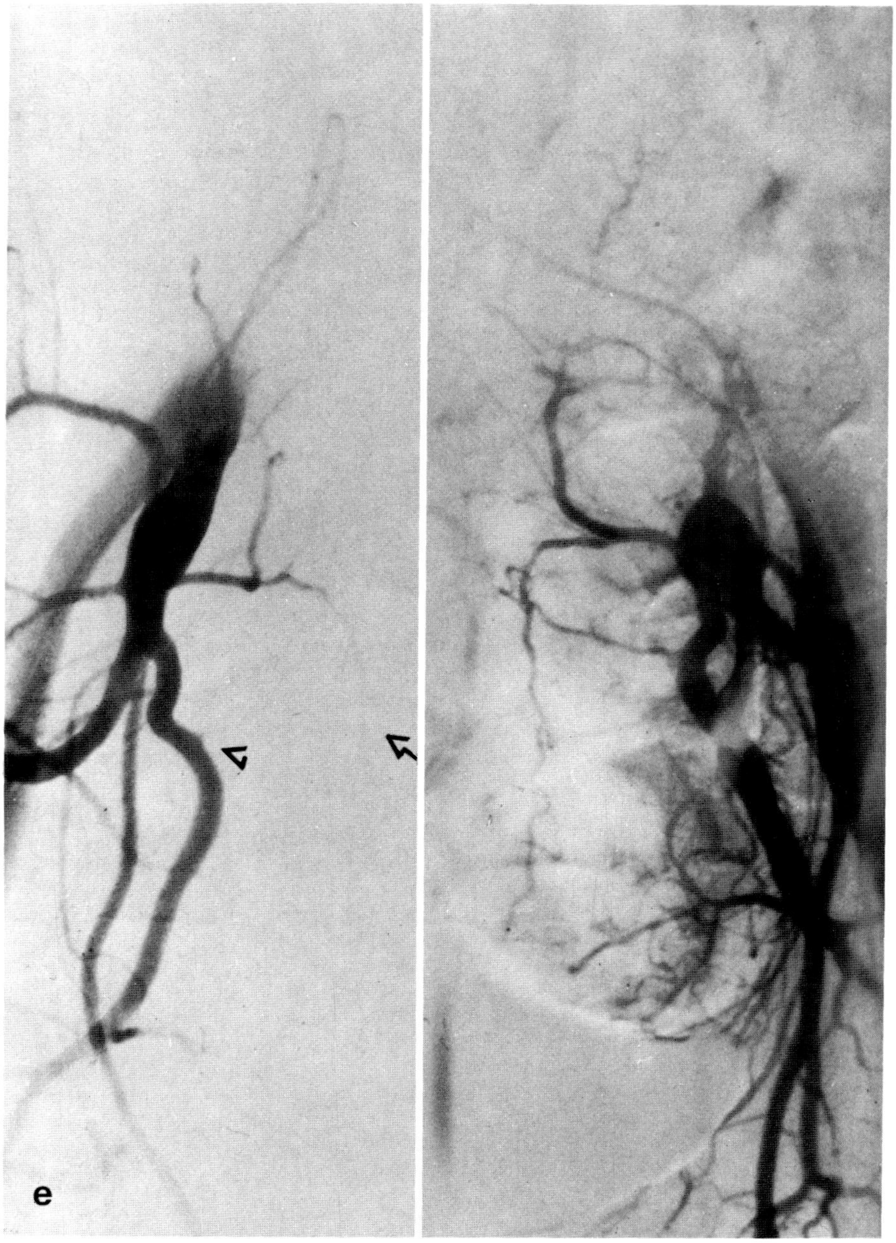

Fig. 92. e After selective embolization of this fistula via the inferior gluteal feeding branch, the paraplegia spectacularly improved

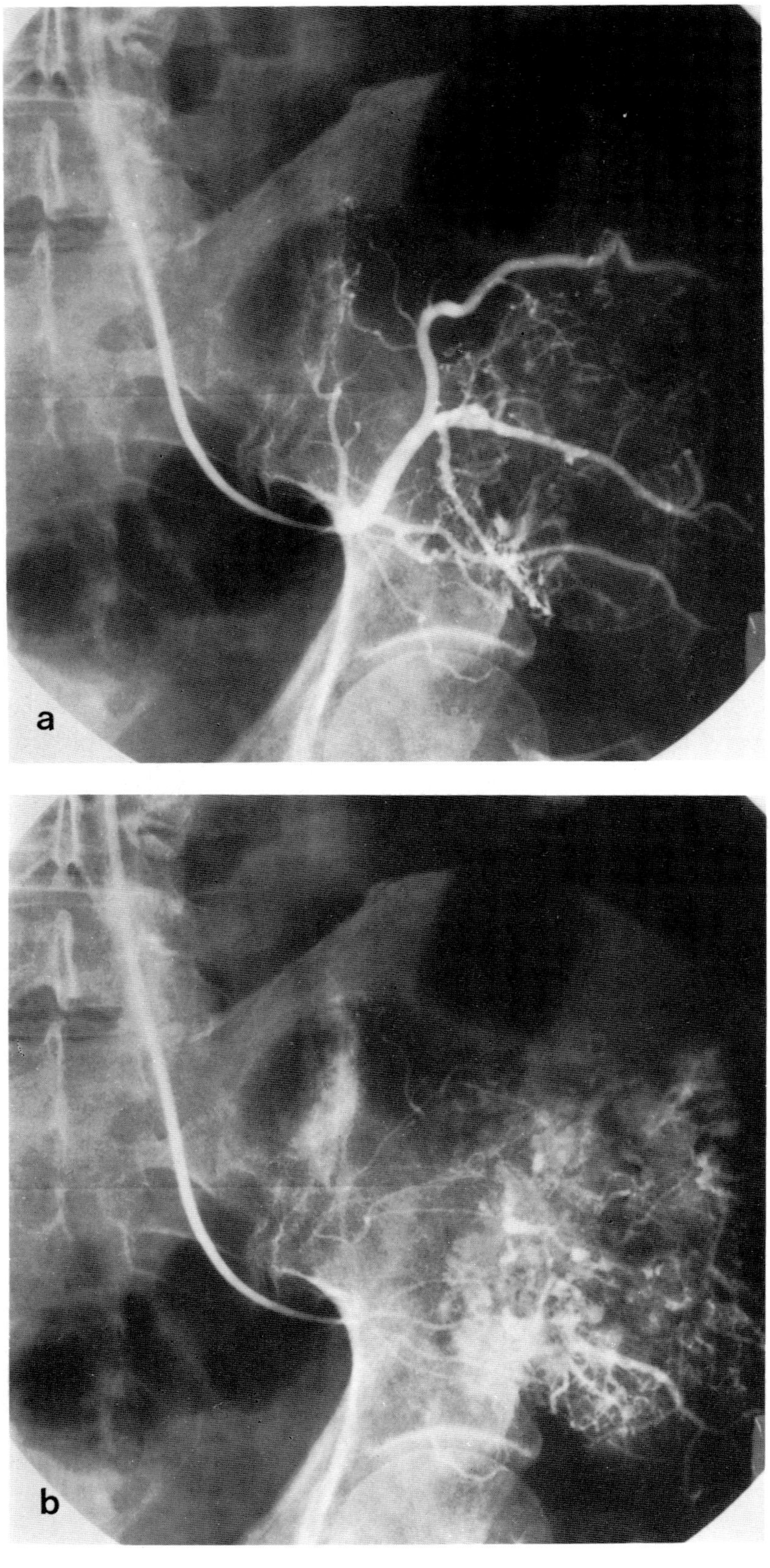
a
b

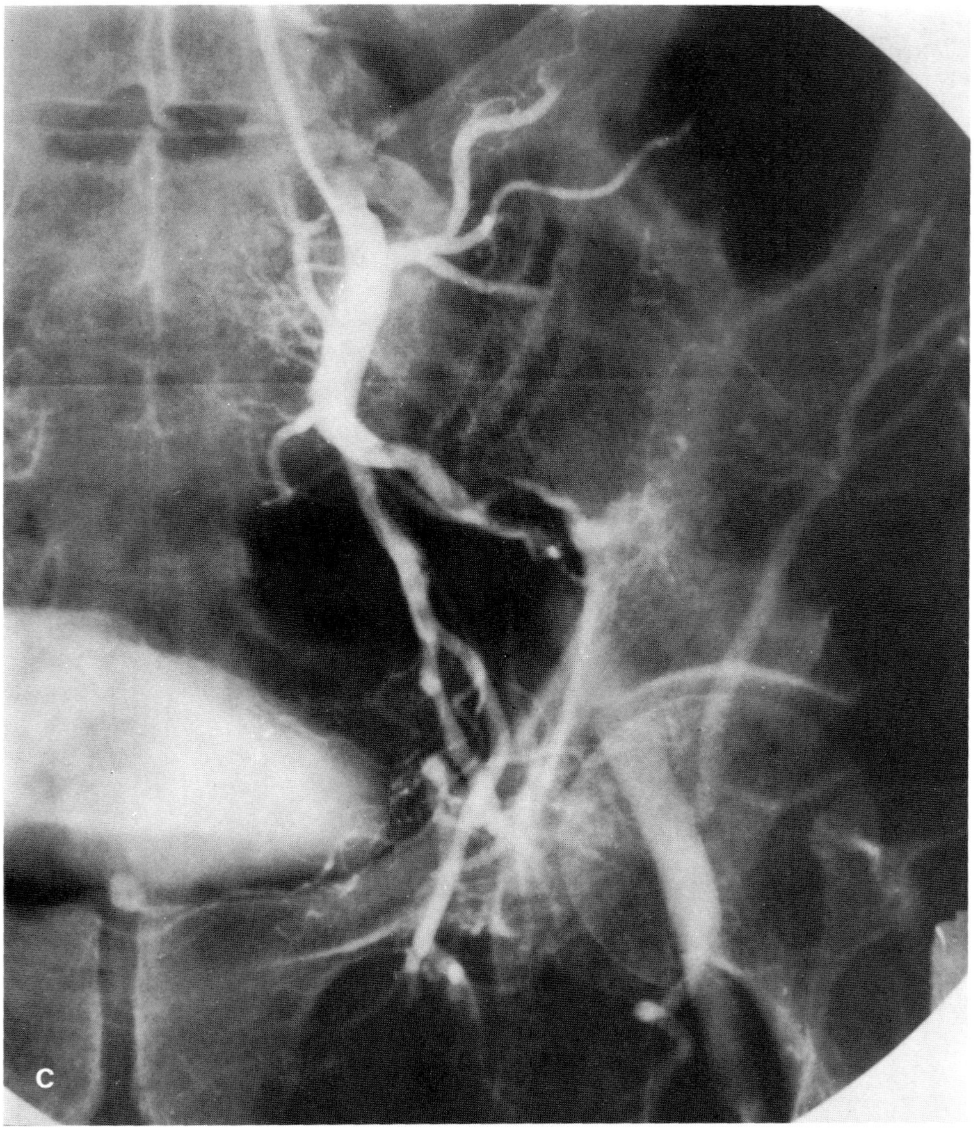

Fig. 93 a–c. Painful iliac bone metastasis from a renal carcinoma. **a** Deep branch of the superior gluteal artery: hypertrophy of the branches and early draining veins. **b** Later phase: venous pools and heterogenous opacification. **c** After embolization of the iliolumbar and superior gluteal arteries, the tumor is no longer opacified by the internal iliac artery, but some feeding branches from the deep circumflex iliac artery remain

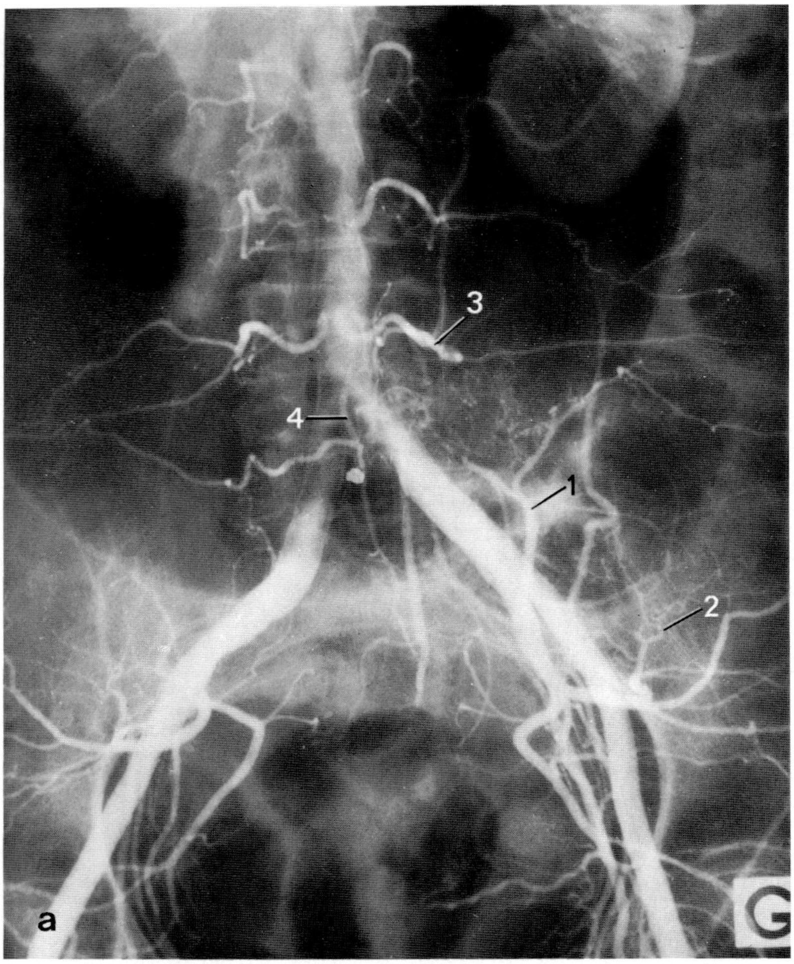
3
4
1
2
a
G

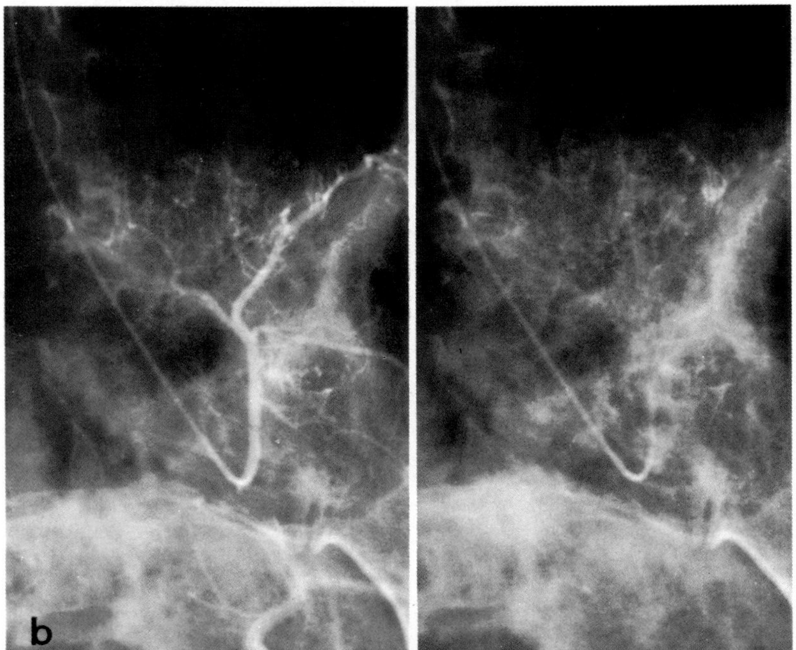
b

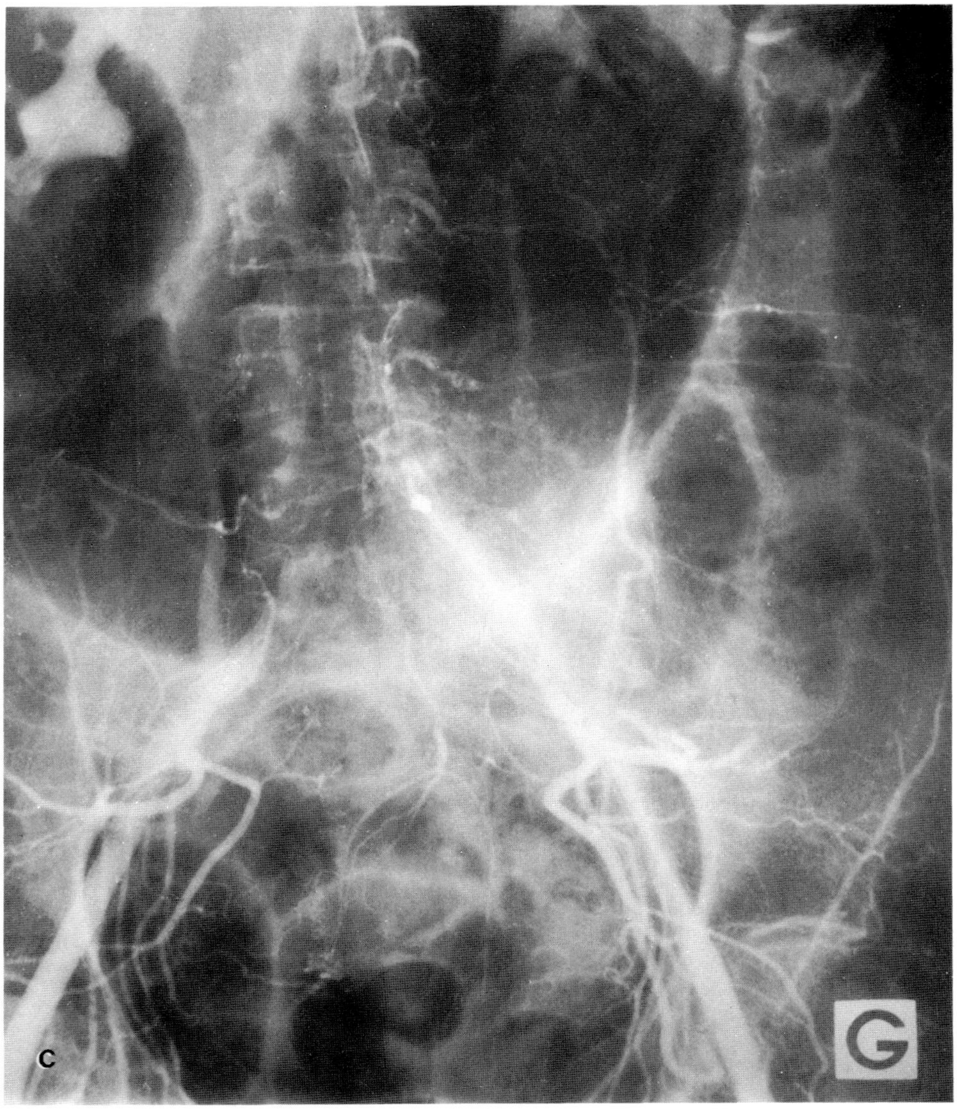

Fig. 94 a–c. 45-year-old woman with left sciatalgias. Sacral chordoma with invasion of the iliac ala and the fifth lumbar vertebra. **a** Aortography: hypervascular tumor fed by the iliolumbar (*1*) superior gluteal (*2*) (internal iliac artery) fourth lumbar and medial sacral arteries (*3* and *4*). **b** Iliolumbar artery. **c** Internal iliac artery; following complete embolization a discrete tumor opacity remains. Successful and bloodless surgical removal

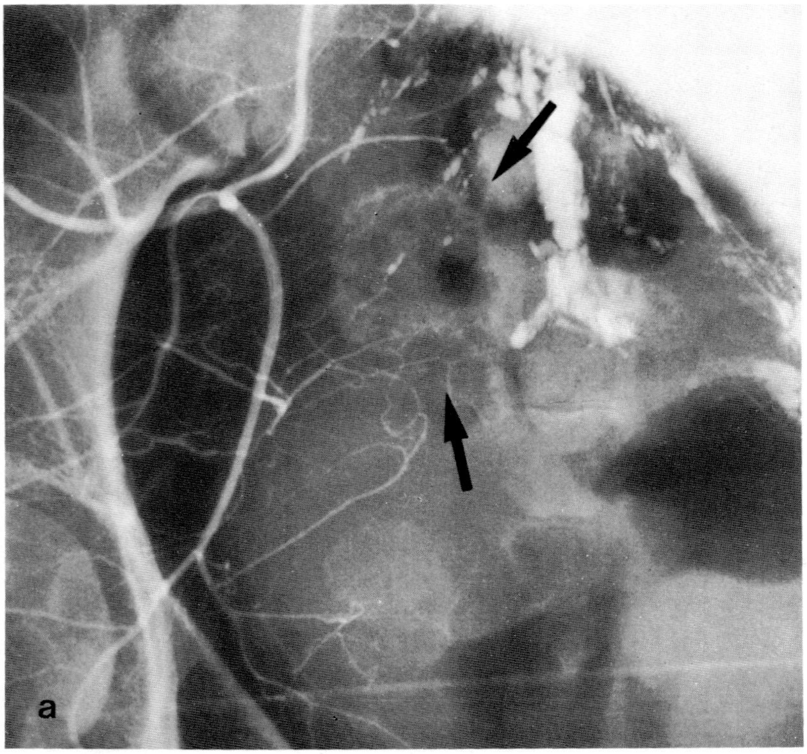
a

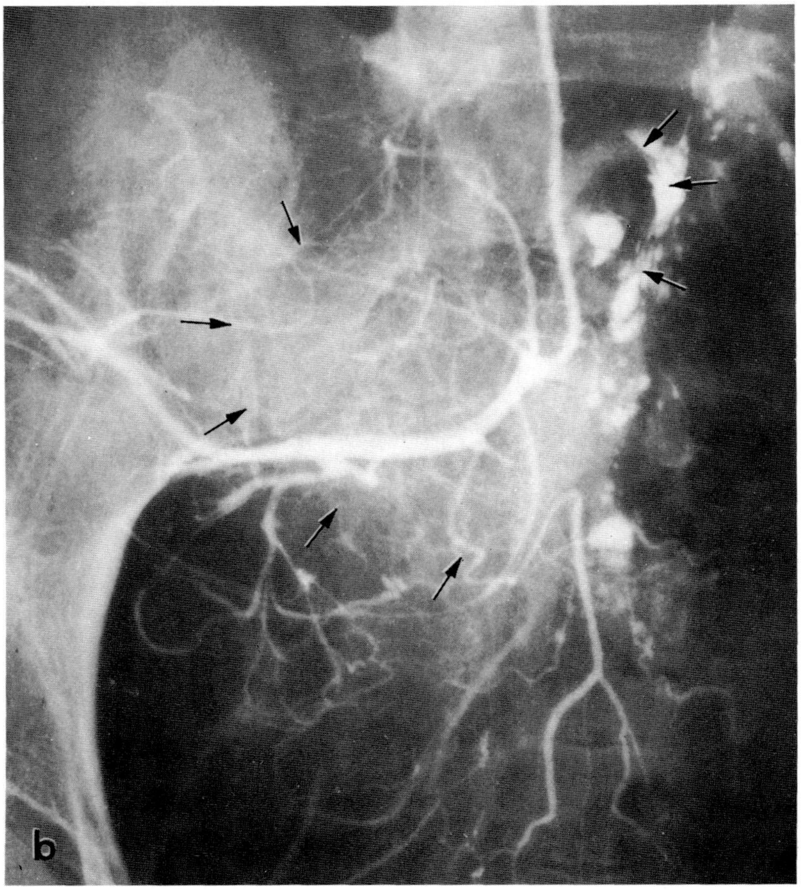
b

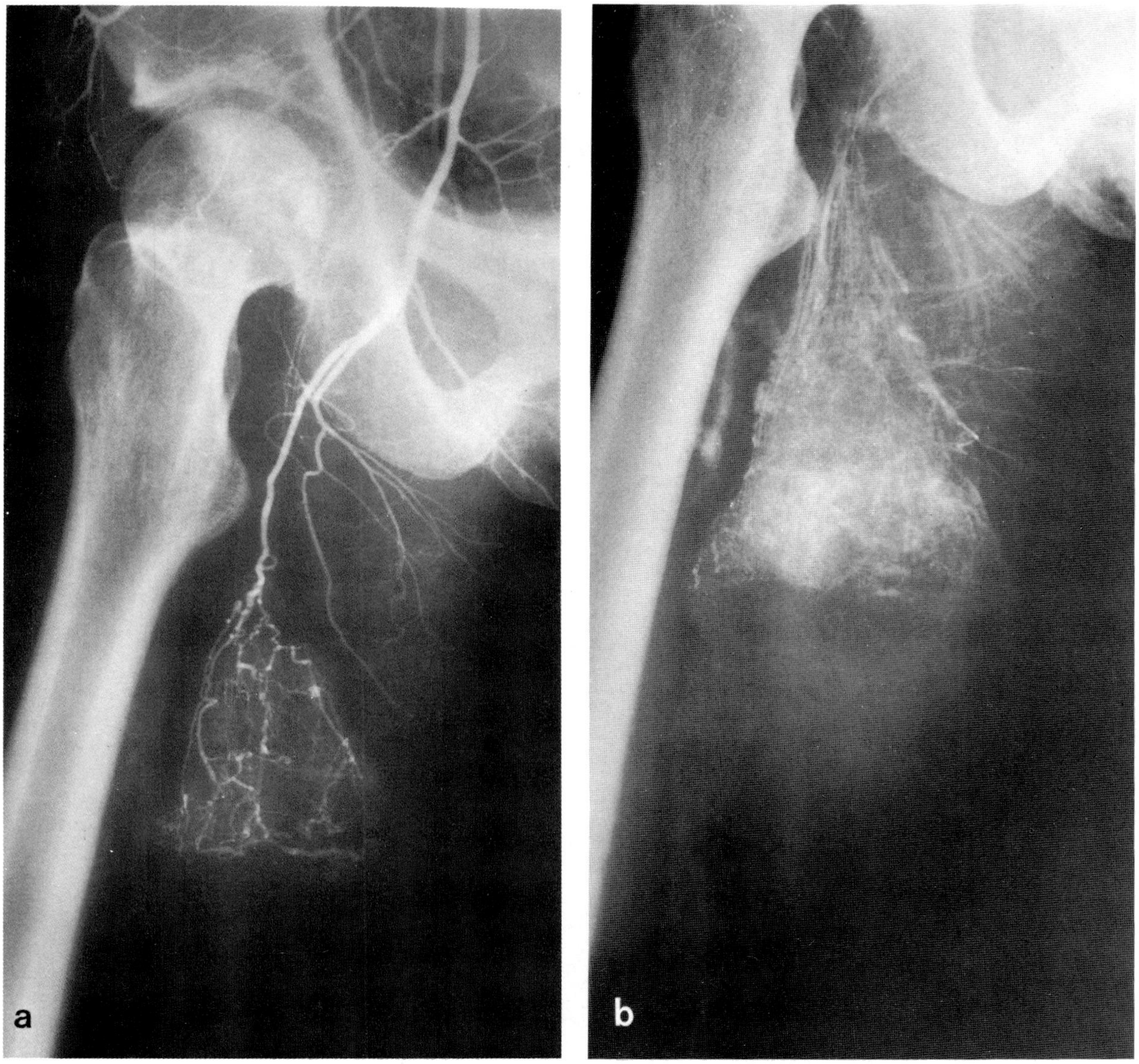

Fig. 96 a, b. Schwannoma of the sciatic nerve. Selective inferior gluteal arteriography opacifies the tumor (by courtesy of Dr. Theron)

◁ **Fig. 95a, b.** Young woman with multiple localizations of Recklinghausen disease and sciatalgia. **a** Internal iliac artery: inferior gluteal artery opacifies a small tumor via the ischiosacral branches (*arrows*). **b, c** One year later recurrence of the tumor and symptomatology: the lesion is very large, extending at the intrapelvic and extrapelvic spaces. There is an extension in the epidural space. *Arrows* show the extensive tumor

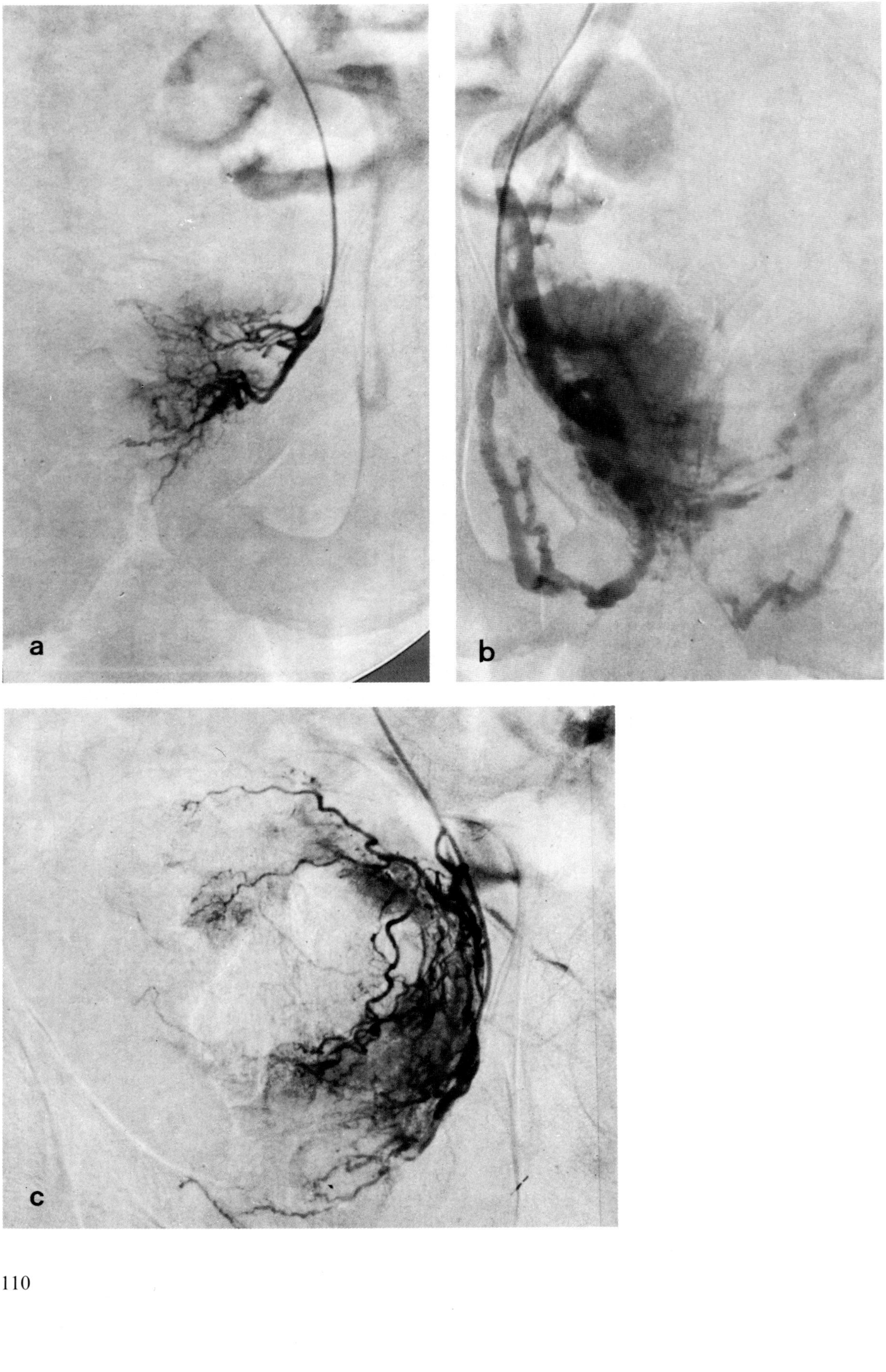
a
b
c

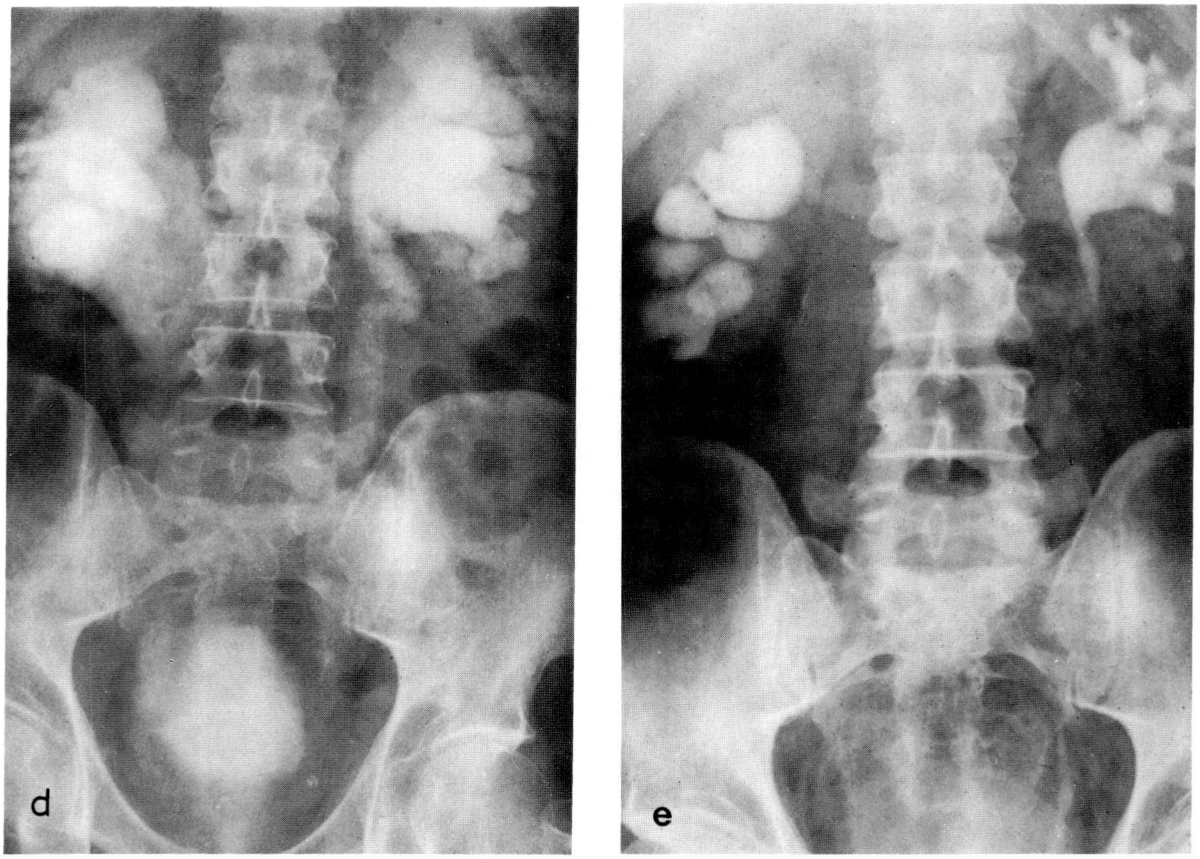

Fig. 97 a–e. Carcinoma of the bladder. Selective inferior vesical arteriography (**a, b**), followed by superior vesical (**c**) arteriography. The embolization diminished hydronephrosis (**d, e**)

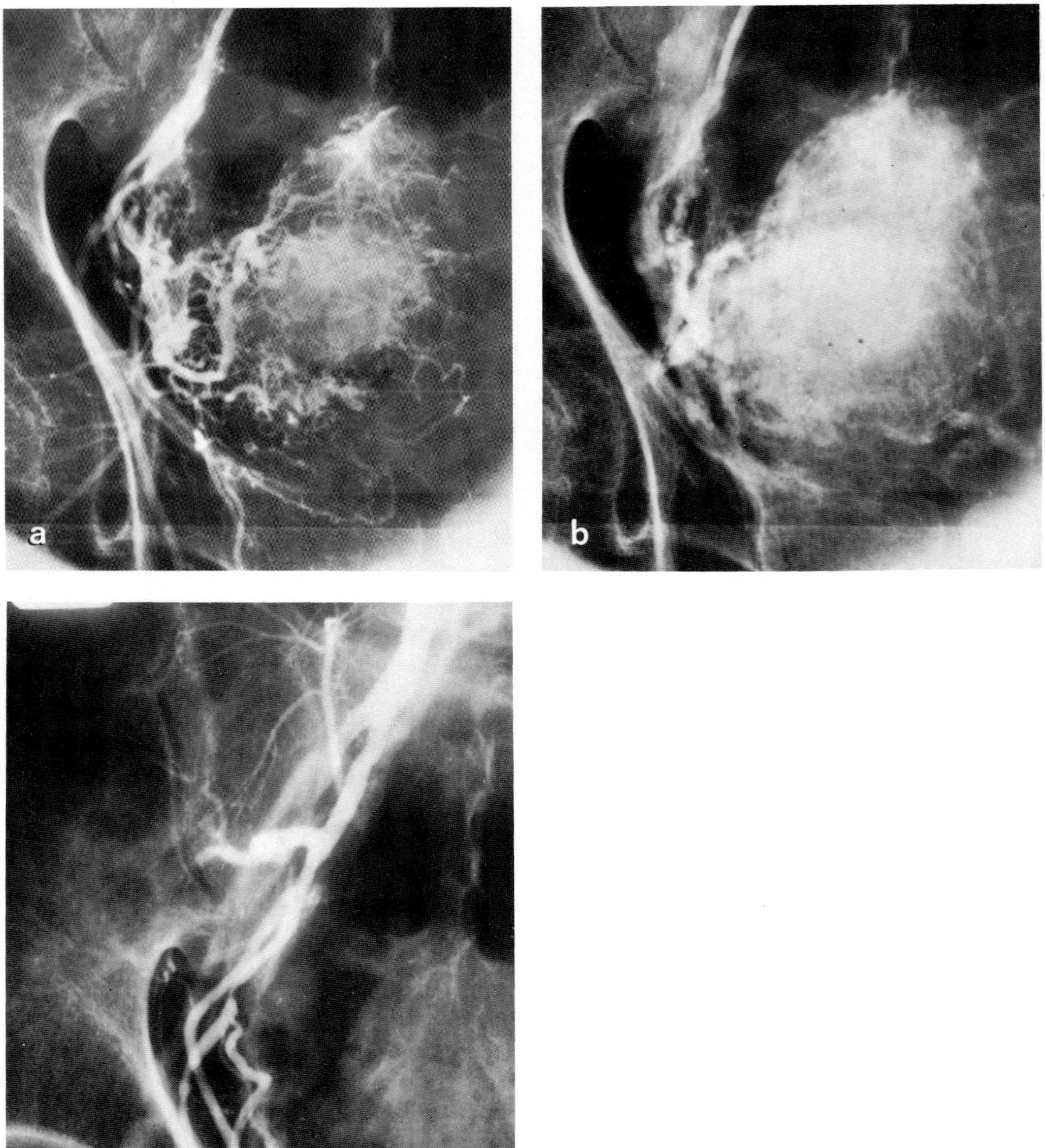
a
b
c

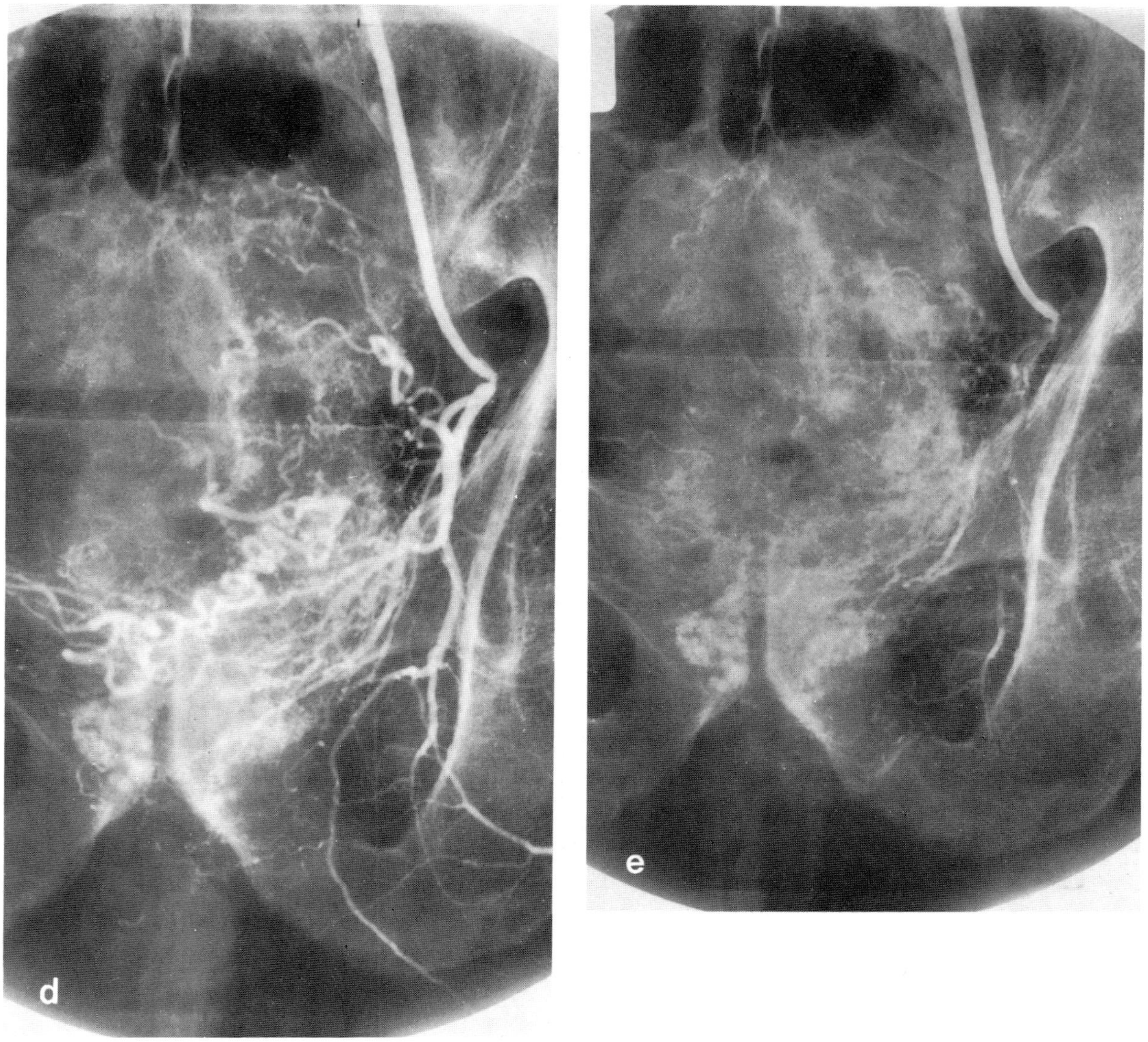

Fig. 98a–e. Diffuse carcinoma of the bladder. Right and left selective arteriography showing diffuse hypervascularization. Successful embolization. Selective right vesical artery (**a, b**) before and after (**c**) embolization; left side (**d**, **e**)

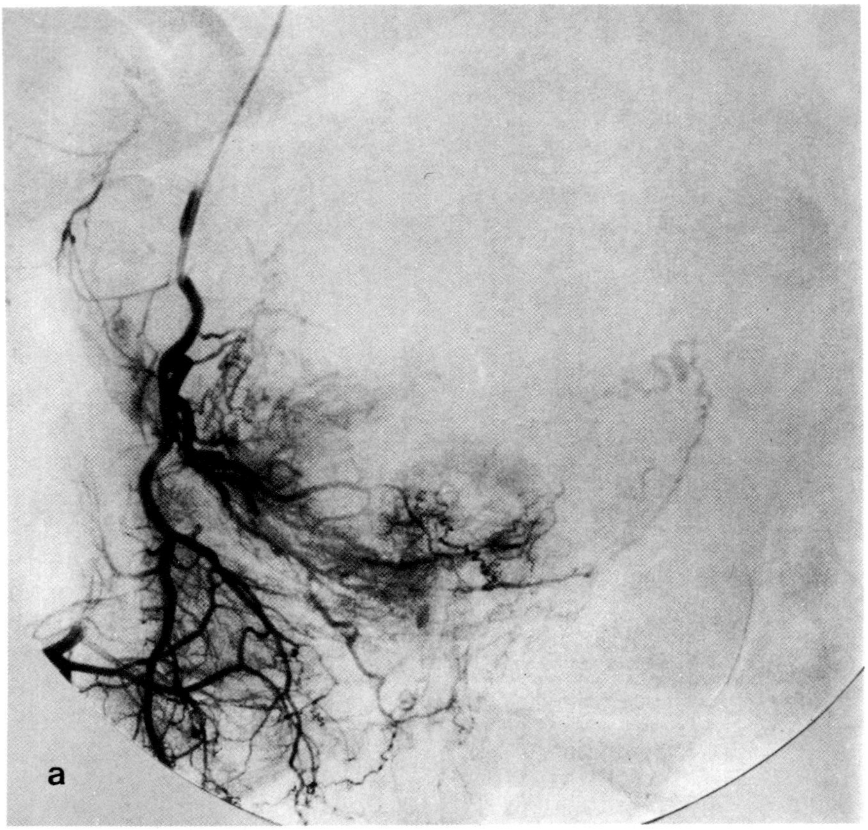
a

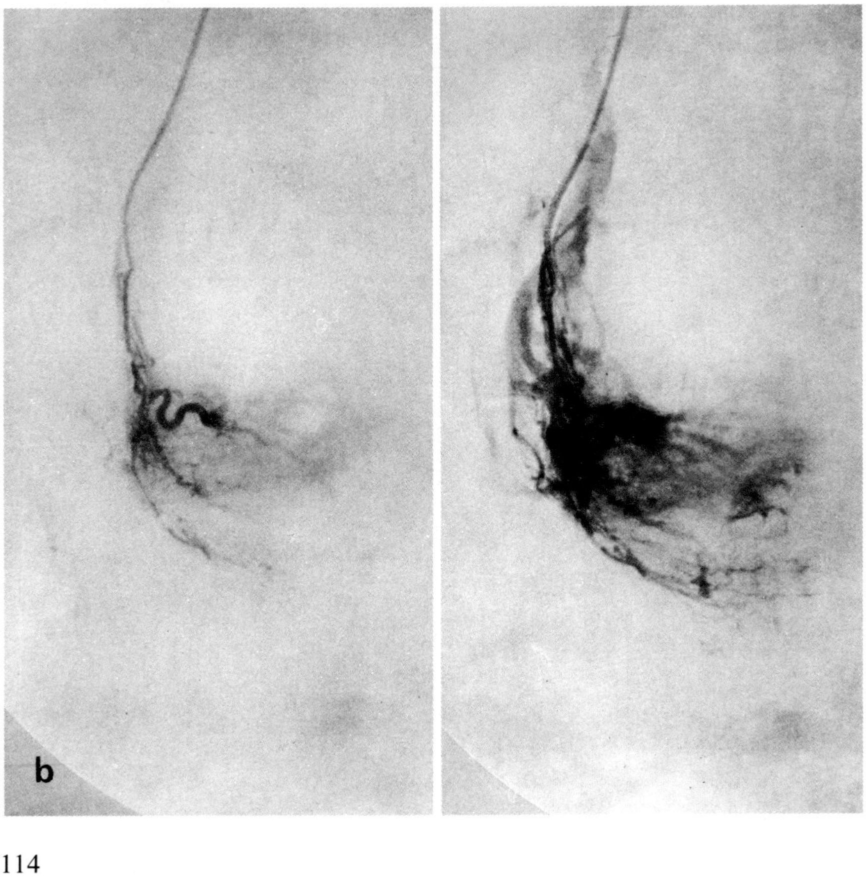
b

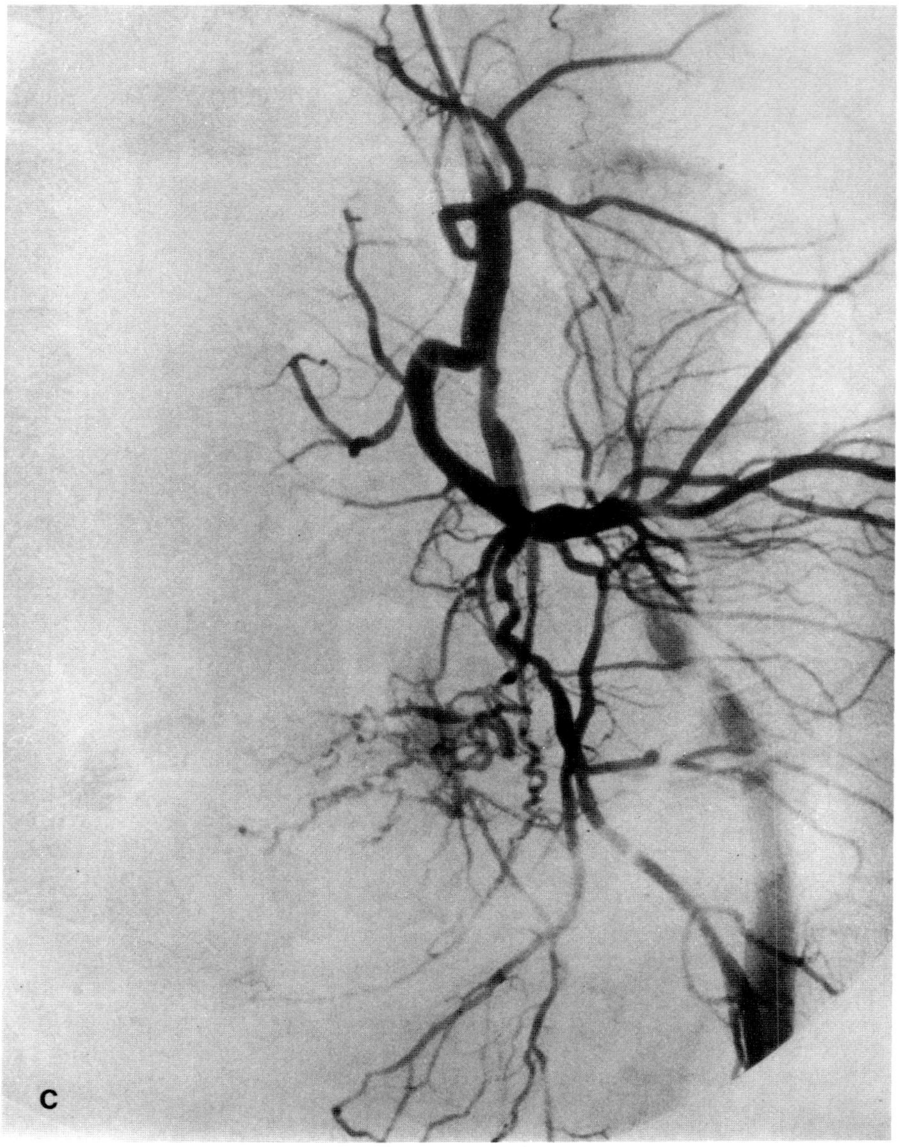

Fig. 99 a–c. Postradiation cystitis with permanent bleeding. Successful embolization. **a** Obturator artery: slight blush on the capillary phase coming from the inferior vesical artery. **b** Superior vesical artery, early and late phases. **c** Contralateral arteriography: irregular, tortuous and narrowed arteries due to irradiation

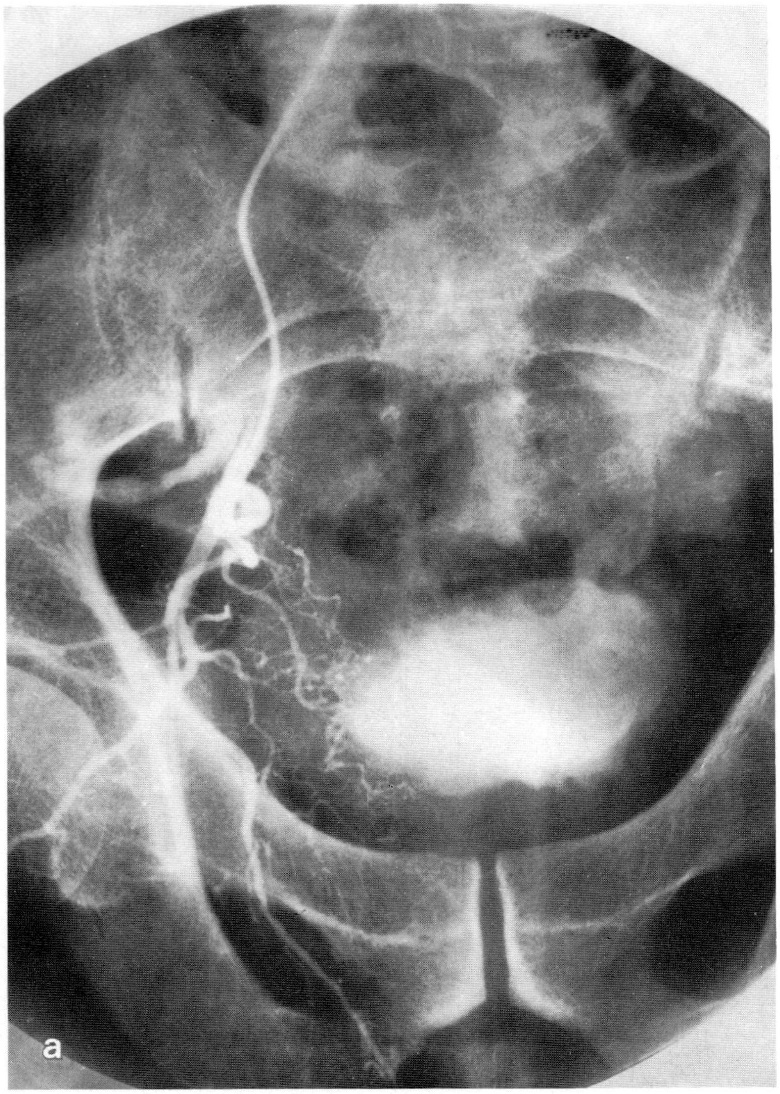

Fig. 100 a–d. Prostatic carcinoma invading the bladder; hemostatic embolization for hemorrhage. Progressive catheterization of the anterior trunk (**a**)

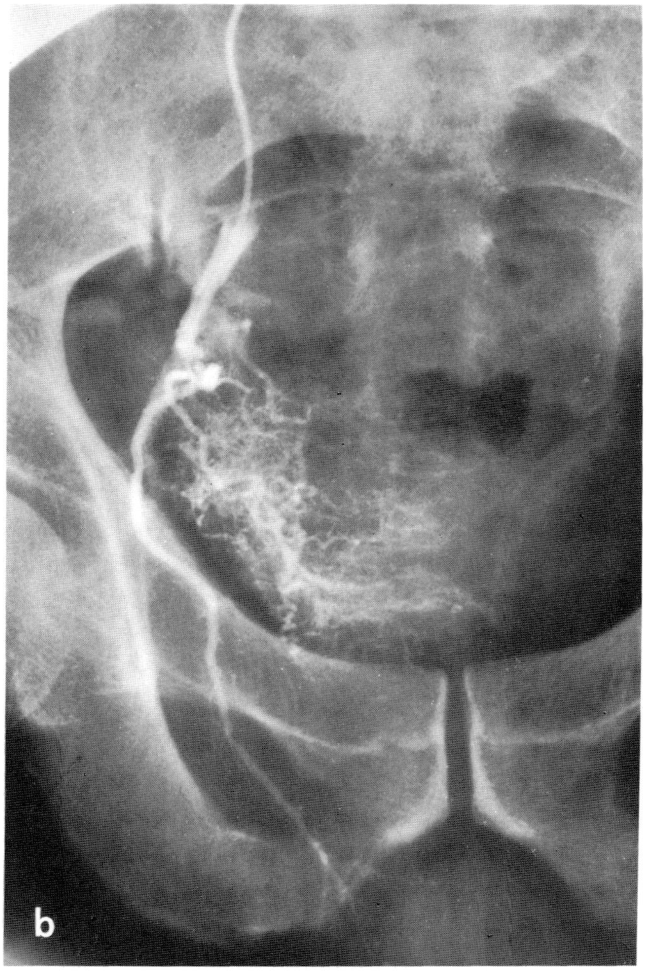

Fig. 100 b–d. Progressive catheterization of the internal pudendal and prostatic arteries, (b) and finally of the c prostatic and d superior vesical arteries

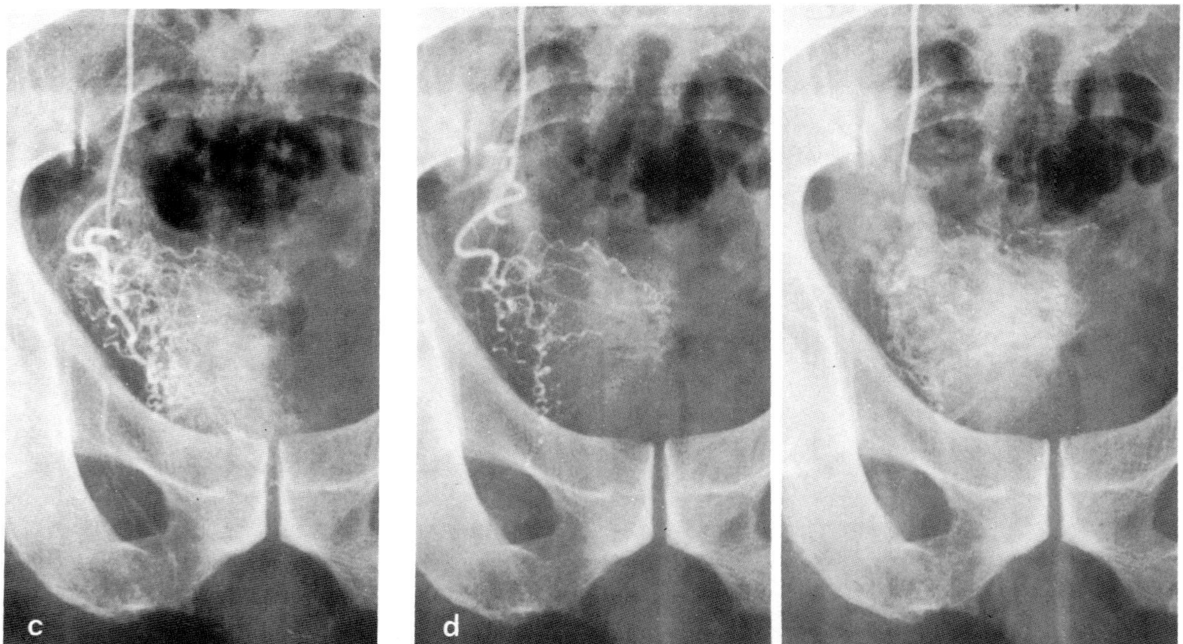

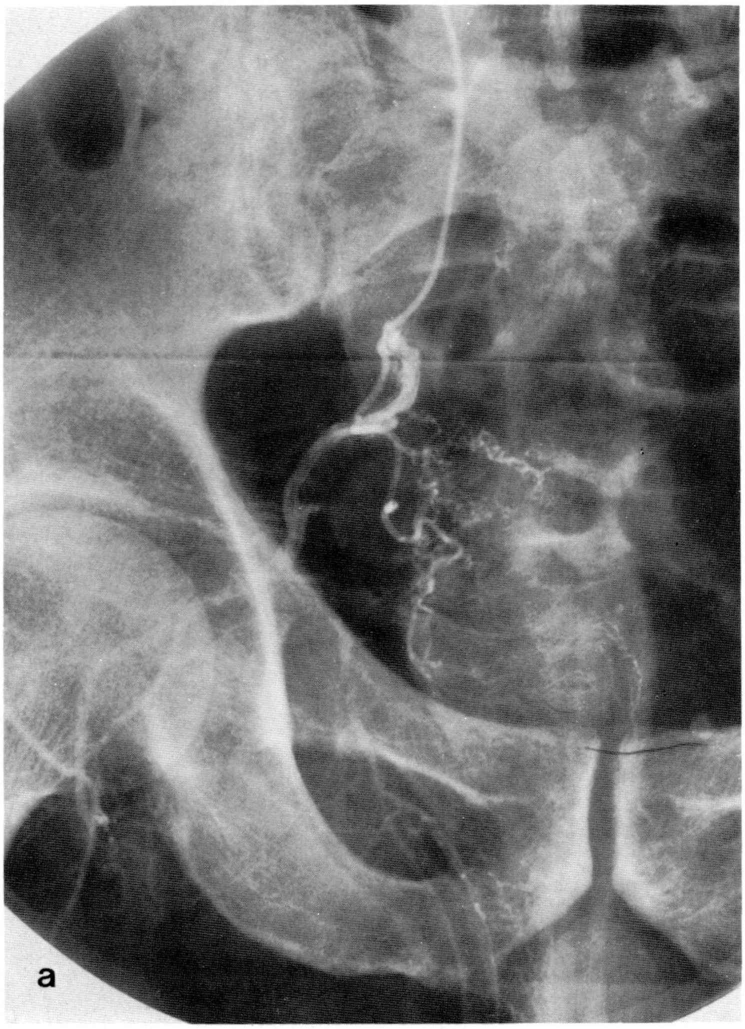

Fig. 101 a, b. Prostatic carcinoma with urinary retention. Reduction in the size of the tumor after embolization.
a Selective opacification of the anterior trunk. **b** Selective opacification of the prostatic artery

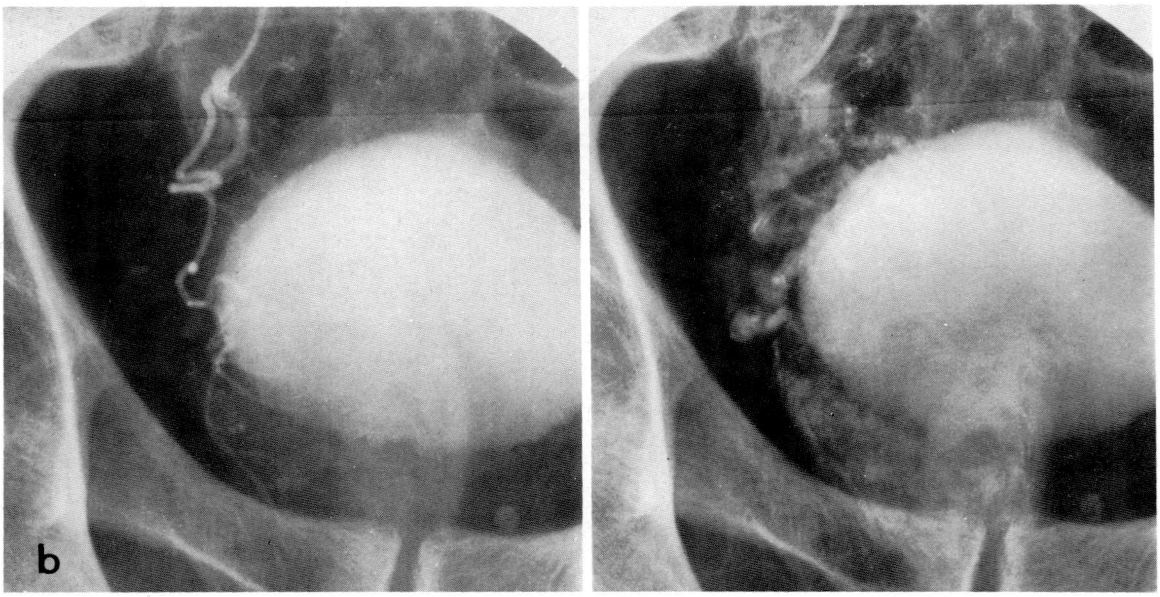

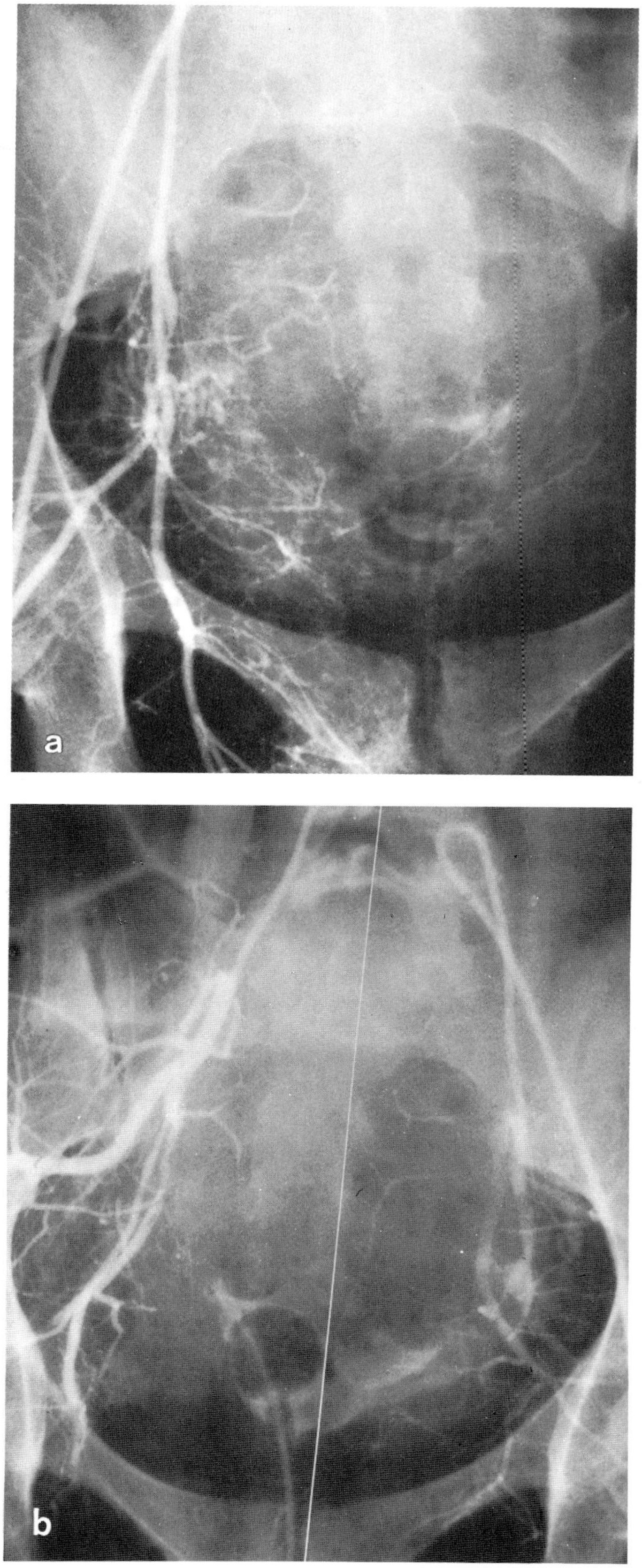

Fig. 102 a, b. Massive postpartum bleeding for which emergency hemostatic hysterectomy would have been the only solution. Emergency arteriography (**a**) and embolization (**b**) successfully stopped the bleeding

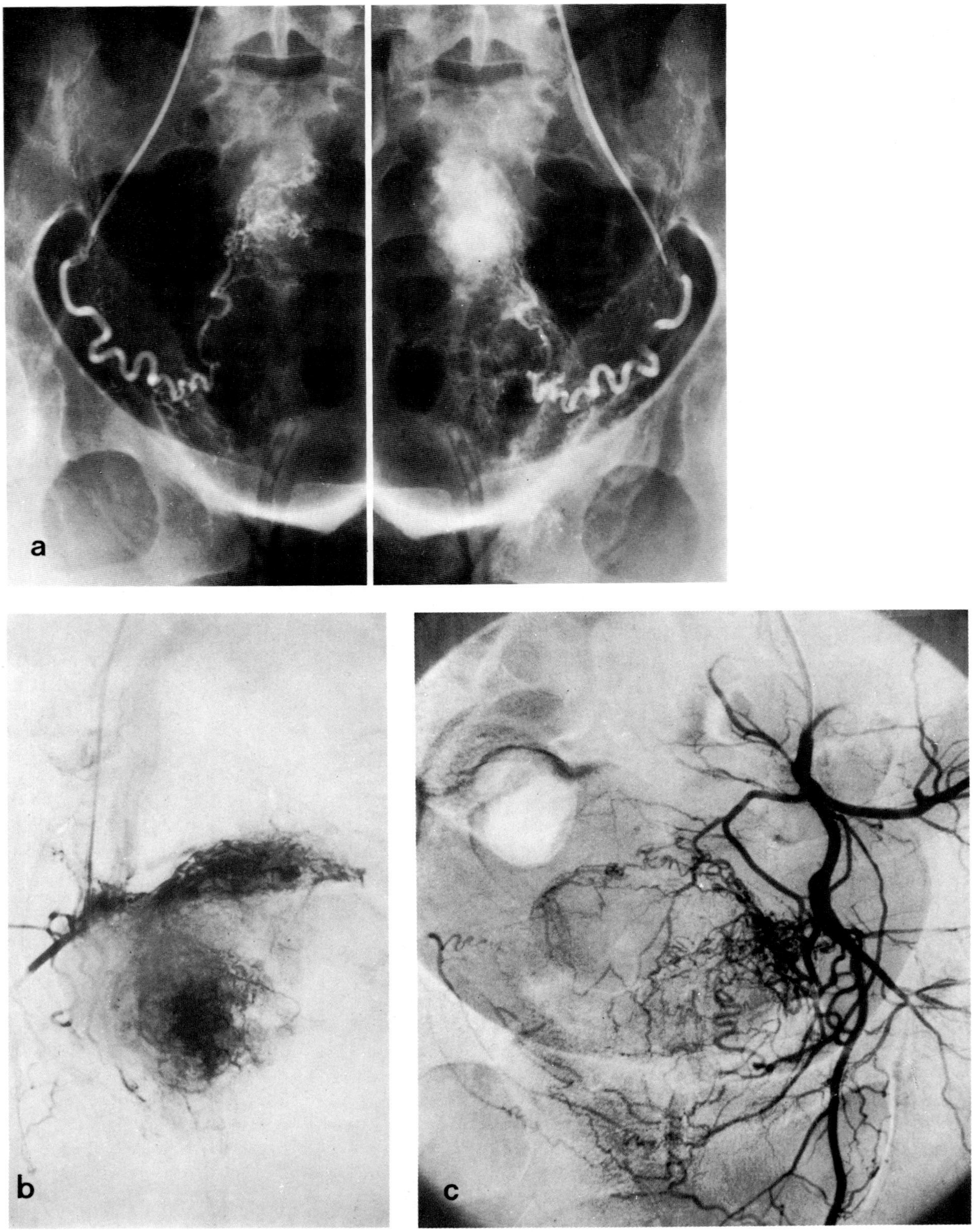

Fig. 103a–f. Invading uterine carcinoma with genital bleeding in an inoperable patient. Hemostatic embolization. Three times: **a** uterine arteries, 6 weeks later; **b, c** accessory arteries, and 3 months later

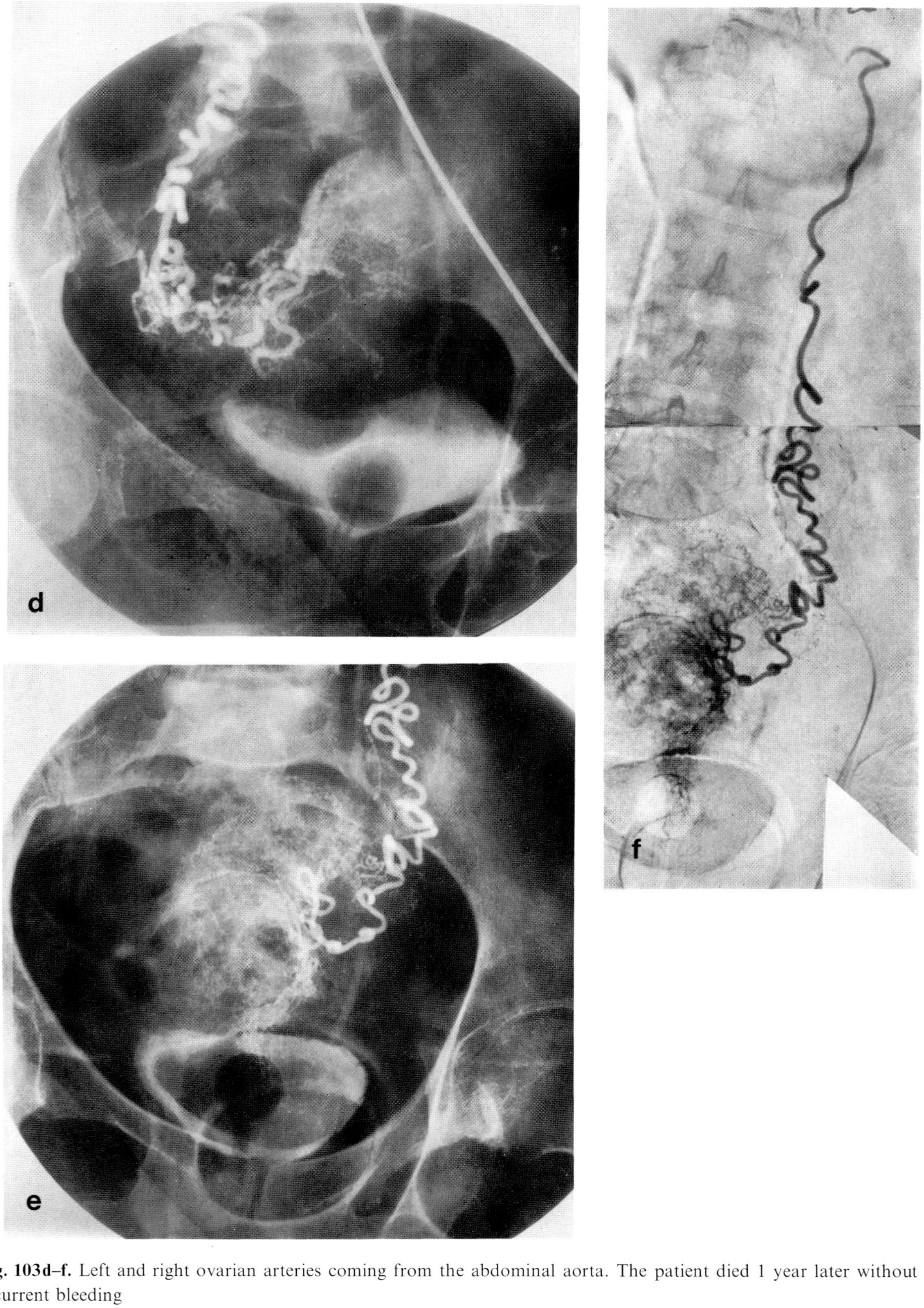

Fig. 103d–f. Left and right ovarian arteries coming from the abdominal aorta. The patient died 1 year later without recurrent bleeding

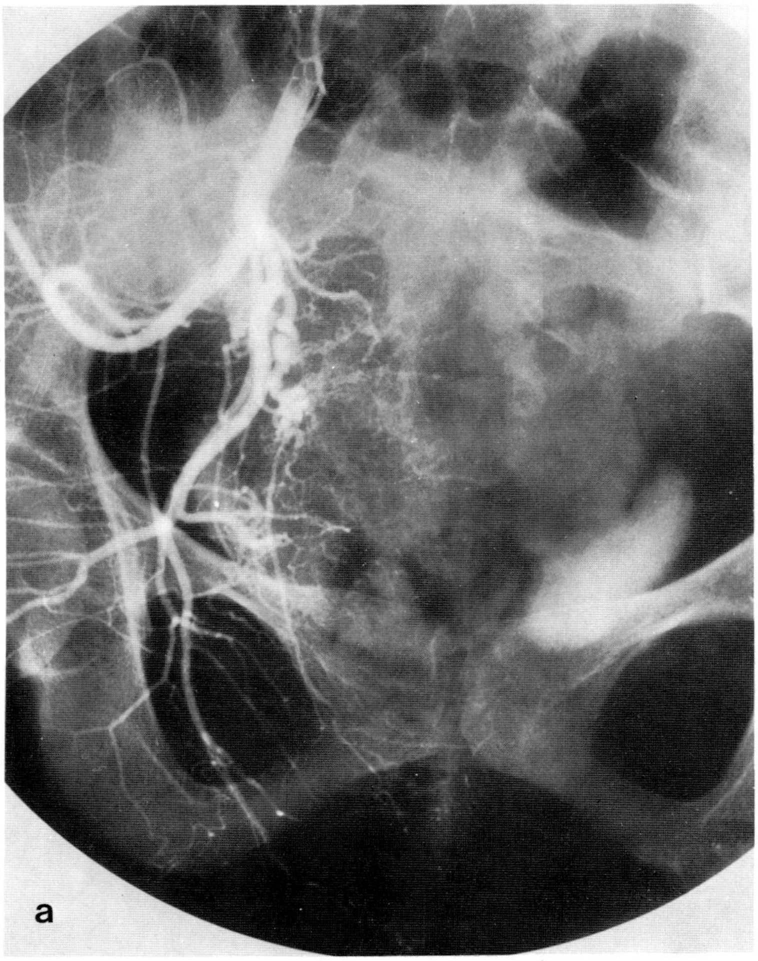
a

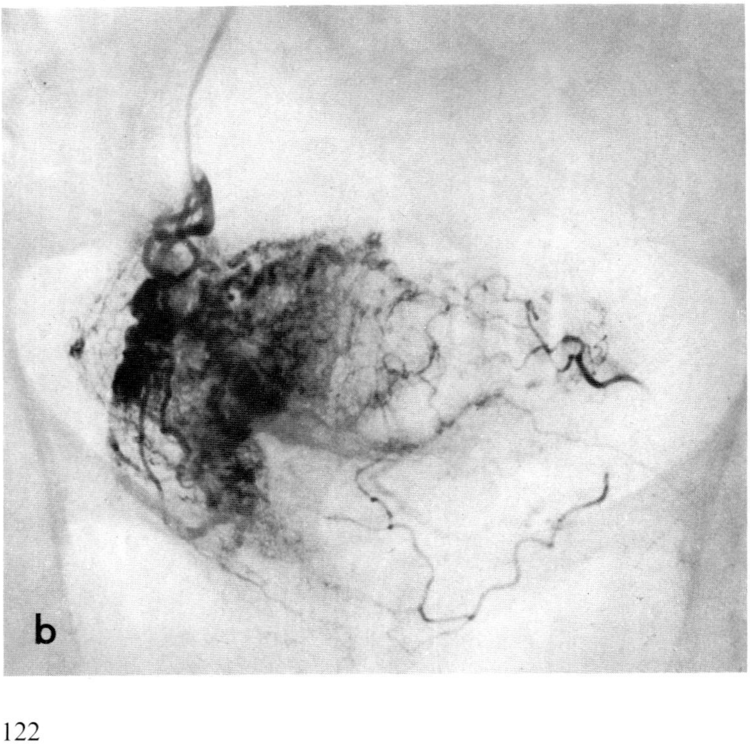
b

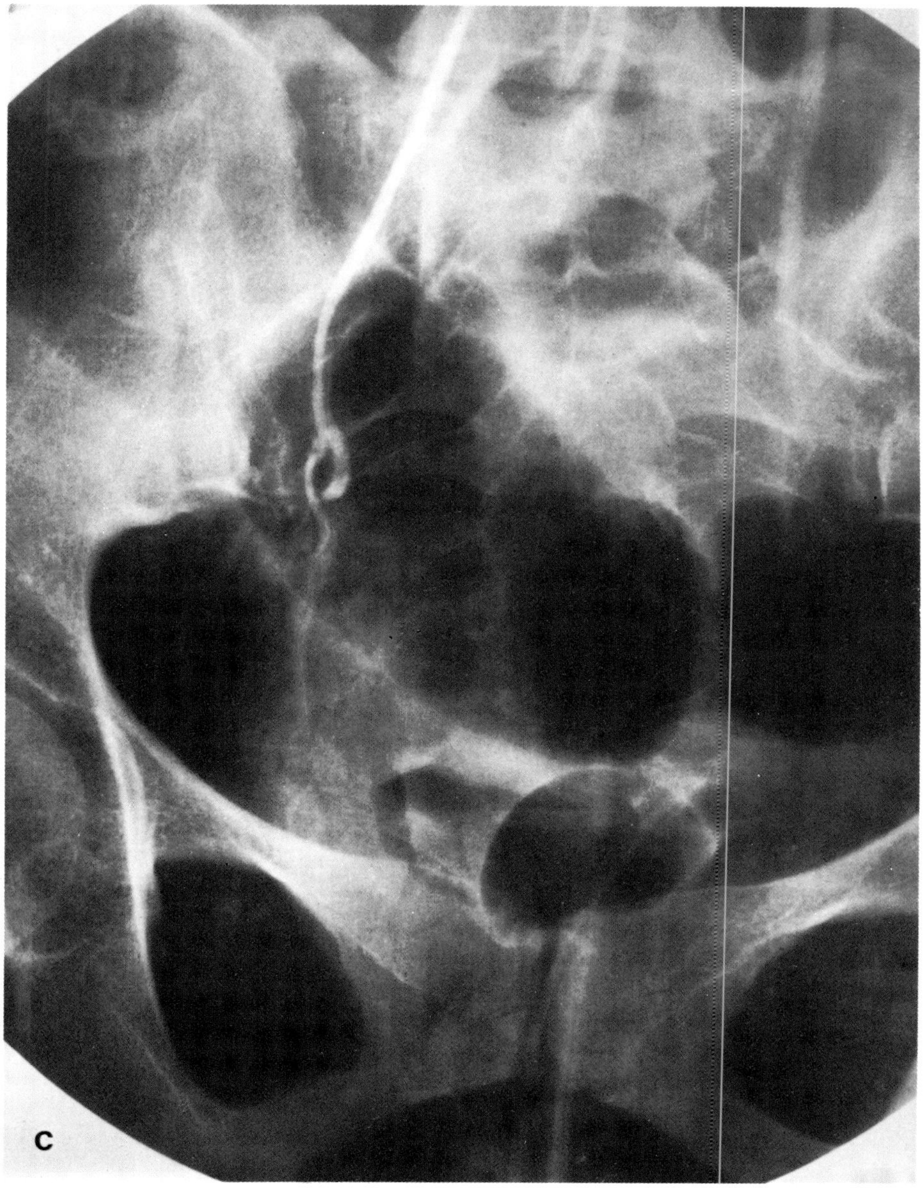

Fig. 104 a–c. Extensive uterine carcinoma with pelvic invasion, pain and hemorrhage. Successful hemostatic embolization. **a** Left internal iliac arteriography: localization of pathologic vessels. **b** Selective catheterization of tumoral vessels. **c** After embolization (the same was performed on the opposite side)

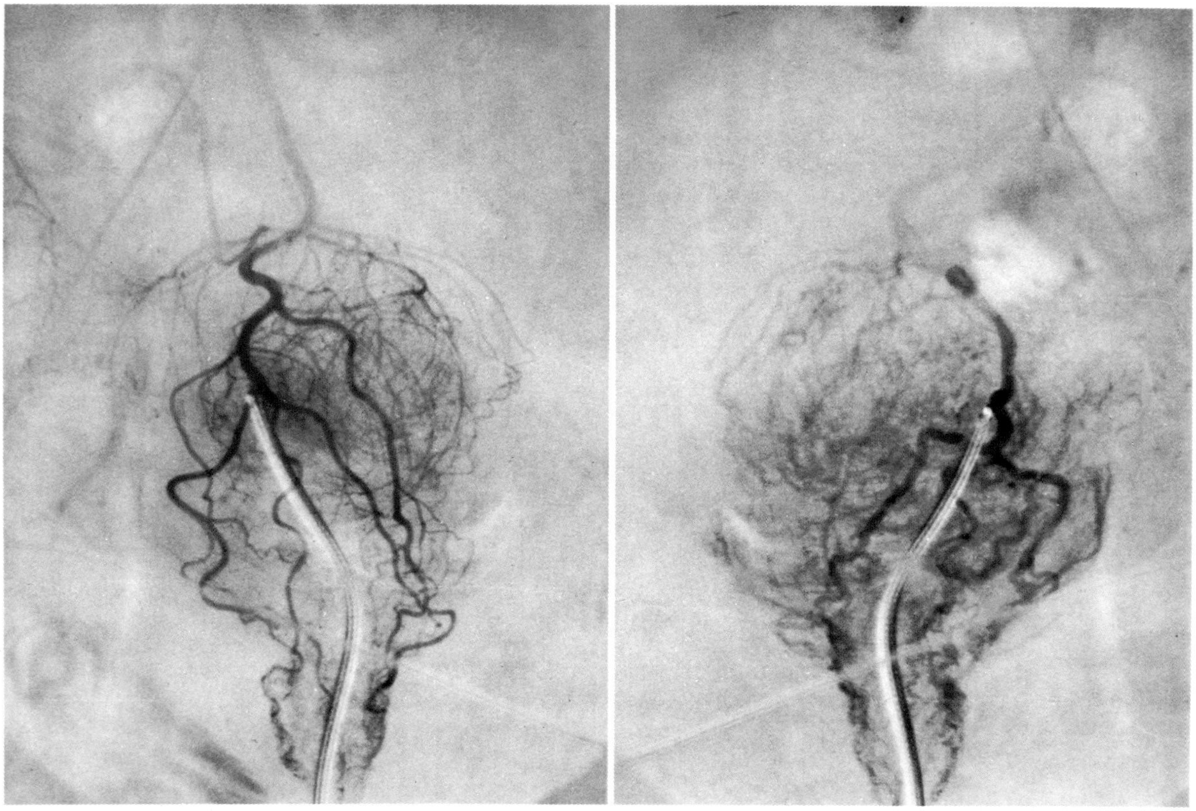

Fig. 105. Postirradiation rectitis associated with chronic bleeding. Arteriography reveals diffuse hypervascularization; embolization successfully stopped the bleeding

5 Bibliography

ADACHI B (1928) Das Arteriensystem der Japaner. Kenkuyusha, Kyoto

ALTEMUS R (1968) Selective catheterization of the hypogastric arteries. Advantages and discussion of technic. Radiology 91/3:484–487

AZZOLINI A (1967) Le lesioni angiodisplasiche del pene; un caso di angioma artero-venose. Minerva Chir 22:974–979

BAKER HL (1960) New approach to percutaneous subclavian angiography. Mayo Clin Proc 35:169–174

BARLOW B, ROTTENBERG RW, SANTULLY TV (1975) Angiographic diagnosis and treatment of bleeding by selective embolization following pelvic fracture in children. J Pediatr Surg 10:939–942

BARTH KH, STRANDBERG JP, WHITE RI (1977) Long term follow up of transcatheter. Embolization with autologous clot, oxycel and gelfoam in domestic swine. Invest Radiol 12/3:273–280

BATTEUR H (1950) Un cas exceptionnel de variation de l'artère obturatrice. CR Assoc Anat (Paris) 11:116–119

BELOU P (1934) Revision anatomica del systema arterial. Ateneo, Buenos Aires

BENNET J, BIGOT R, DOYON D 61962) Techniques d'exploration radiologique de l'aorte et ses branches. EMC (Radiodiagn) 3:32 210 $A^{10}{}_{\alpha}C^{50}$

BENVENTI FA, NOBACK GJ (1949) Distribution of the blood vessels of the prostate and urinary bladder; application to retropubic prostatectomy. J Urol 62/5:663–671

BERTI-RIBOLI EP, CERRUTI GB, MALCHIODI C, REGGIANI G (1957) Studio angiografico dei tumori vescicali. Minerva Urol 9:10–18

BEZZI E, MACALUSO G 61957) Contributo alla diagnosi dell cancero della prostata. Prezentazione di un methodo arteriografico. Bull Soc Piem Chir 27:84–102

BOBBIO A, BEZZI E, ROSSI L (1959) Pelvic angiography in diseases of the prostatic gland. AJR 82/5:784–792

BOIJSEN E, NILSSON J (1962) Angiography in the diagnosis of tumors of the urinary bladder. Acta Radiol (Stockh) 57:241–258

BOLLACK C, SUWCER A, JURSCHEK F (1966) A propos d'un cas rare d'hémangiome caverneux de la vessie. J Urol Nephrol (Paris) 72:171–177

BONTE G, DESRUELLES J, SALEMBIER Y (1954) Atlas d'aortographie abdominale. Expansion Scientifique, Paris

BORELL U, FERNSTROM I (1953) The adnexal branches of the uterine artery. An arteriographic study in human subjects. Acta Radiol (Stockh) 40:561

BORELL U, FERNSTROM I, LINDBLOM K, WESTMAN A (1952) The diagnostic value of arteriography of the iliac artery in gynecology and obstetrics. Acta Radiol (Stockh) 38:247–263

BOTTOMLEY JP, WHITEHOUSE GH (1975) Congenital arteriovenous malformations of the uterus demonstrated by angiography. Acta Radiol (Stockh) 16/1:43–48

BOUISSOU H, TALAZAC A (1958) Vascularisation artérielle intraparenchymateuse de la prostate. CR Assoc Anat (Paris) 45:199–203

BOURGERY J (1836) Traité complet de l'anatomie de l'homme. Delaunay, Paris

BOXALL TA, SMART PJG, GRIFFITHS JD (1963) The blood supply of the distal segment of the rectum in anterior resection. Br J Surg 50/222:399–404

Braibanti T, Rossi L, Gagnoni G, Shippisi (1965) L'arteriographica pelvica. Minerva Medica, Turin

Braithwaite JL (1952) The arterial supply of the male urinary bladder. Br J Urol 24/1:64–71

Braithwaite JL (1953) The effects of ligation of the pelvic arteries on the viability of the urinary bladder and the sufficiency of the collateral circulation in the experimental animal. Br J Surg 40/164:610–616

Brault B, Marsault C, Moulin JD (1976) Embolisation arterielle dans le traitement des metrorragies d'origine tumorale.Nouv Presse Med 5/6:1043–1046

Braunstein PW, Skudder PA, MacCarroll JR (1964) Concealed hemorrhage due to pelvic fracture. J Traum 4:832–838

Bron KM (1966) Selective visceral and total abdominal arteriography via the left axillary artery in the older age group. AJR 97/2:432–437

Cerf L (1896) Les vaisseaux sanguins du périnée et des viscères pelviens. Medical dissertation, University of Paris

Chait A, Moltz A, Nelson JH Jr (1968) The collateral arterial circulation in the pelvis. AJR 102/2:392–400

Champetier J, Charignon G, Durand A, Letoublon C, Marty F, Guignier M (1977) Interest and limits of arteriography in one case of abdomino-pelvic trauma. J Chir (Paris) 113/3:59–66

Chevrier LE (1955) Etude anatomique des artères de la vessie. Applications à la chirurgie plastique de cet organe. Medical dissertation, University of Paris

Chiras J, Roche A, Curet P, Merland JJ, Doyon D (1980) Pelvic embolization in uterine neoplasms. Bull Cancer 69/1:107–108

Clegg EJ (1955) The arterial supply of the human prostate and seminal vesicles. J Anat 89/2:209–217

Cordier C, Chatain Y (1950) Les pédicules chirurgicaux des organes pelviens. CR Assoc Anat (Paris)

Cornell SH (1967) Angiography in the staging of bladder carcinoma. J Iowa Med Soc 57:331–335

Dadie A (1966) Considérations sur l'artère hypogastrique du nouveauné africain de Côte d'Ivoire. Medical dissertation, University of Paris

Dubreuil-Chambardel L (1923) Notes sur la persistance de l'artère. Combilicale chez l'adulte. Arch Anat Anthropol 8:349–352

Duclaux M (1902) Anomalies de l'épigastrique et de l'obturatrice. Bull Anat (Paris) 4:58–59

Duclos JM, Chanzy M, Alexandre JH, Barin F (1972) Contribution à l'étude de la vascularisation prostatique. Arch Anat Pathol 20/4:355–358

Dufour M, Rigaud A, Gouaze A (1951) Variations du mode de division du tronc de l'artère hypogastrique en fonction du sexe. CR Assoc Anat (Paris) 4:449–457

Esguerra A, Carjaval A, Mouton E (1973) Pelvic arteriography in the diagnosis of hemangioma of the bladder. J Urol 109/4:609–611

Faller A, Widmer O (1955) Contribution à l'artériographie du rectum. In: VI° Congrès, Fed Int Anat. Masson, Paris, pp 69–70

Farabeuf A (1905) Les vaisseaux sanguins des organes génito-urinaires du périnée et du pelvis. Masson, Paris

Fernstrom I (1955) Arteriography of the uterine artery. Acta Radiol [Suppl] (Stockh) 122:1–128

Finterty JC (1949) Persistent ischiatic artery. Anat Rec 97:597–595

Fischer G, Colon J, Mayer M, Dargent M (1966) Intérêt de l'artériographie au cours de la chimiothérapie intra-artérielle des cancers. Première partie: cancers pelviens. Ann Radiol (Paris) 9:367–376

Geller G (1970) Techniques d'angiographie sélective de l'artère iliaque interne. Radiol Clin Biol (Basel) 39:4–3, 180–182

Gerard G (1913) Sur les variations d'origine et de nombre des artères génitales internes de l'homme. Bibl Anat 23:206–220

Gilis P (1902) Le tronc de l'artère hypogastrique. Nouv Montpellier Med 14:1–2

Goldstein HM, Medellin H, Ben Menachem Y, Wallace S (1975) Transcathteter arterial embolization in the management of bleeding in the cancer patient. Radiology 115:603–608

Goerttler V (1977) Prostatic gland arteriography. Vascular supply, diagnosis and differential diagnosis of adenoma and carcinoma of the prostate. Radiology 17/6:256–262

Gouaze A (1951) Le système artériel hypogastrique (influence du squelette du bassin). Medical dissertation, University of Bordeaux

Gouaze A, Sentenac M, Odano R (1956) Contribution à l'étude de l'irrigation artérielle de la prostate. CR Assoc Anat (Paris) 43:374–381

Gouaze A, Odano R, Chantepie C (1957a) Contribution à l'étude de la vascularisation artérielle de la vessie. CR Assoc Anat (Paris) 44:331–340

Gouaze A, Odano R, Chantepie G (1957b) A propos des artères des vésicules séminales et du canal déférent. Soc Anat Paris

Gouverneur R, Garcin A (1924) Etude radiographique de la vascularisation vésicale. Etude et Mémoires Soc Anat Paris 21:184

Haldt T, Mygind T (1974) Control of life-threatening vesical hemorrhage by unilateral hypogastric artery muscle embolization. J Urol 122:60–63

Heaston DK, Mineau DE, Brown BT, Miller FJ (1979) Transcatheter arterial embolization for control of persistent massive peerperal hemorrhage after bilateral surgical hypogastric artery ligation. AJR 133:152–154

Heindel CC, Dugger GS, Guinto FC (1975) Spinal arteriovenous malformation with hypogastric blood supply. Case report. J Neurosurg 42/4 :462–464

Higgins CB, Bookstein JJ, Davis GB, Galloway DC, Barr JW (1977) Therapeutic embolization for intractable chronic bleeding. Radiology 122:473–478

Jatschinski S (1891) Die typischen Verzweigungsformen der arteria hypogastrica. Int Monatsschr Anat Phys 8:114

Kerr WS, Margolies MN, Ring EJ, Waltman AC, Baum SN (1973) Arteriography in pelvic fractures with massive hemorrhage. J Urol 109:479–482

Kiss F (1947) Les vaisseaux sanguins de la prostate. Acta Anat (Basel) 4:155–160

Kosinski C (1929) Sur la ramification des artères iliaques. CR Assoc Anat (Paris) 316–335

Kuss R, Bories J, Merland JJ, Marsault C, Le Guillou M (1974) Quelques possibilités d'embolisation en urologie. J Urol Nephrol (Paris) 10/11:845–852

Lacy S, Whitley JE, Cox CE (1972) Vesical arteriography: an adjunct to staging of bladder tumors. Br J Urol 42 50–55

Lang EK (1963) Use of arteriography in the demonstration and staging of bladder tumors. Radiology 80:62–68

Lang EK (1967) Arteriography in gynecology. Radiol Clin North Am 5:133–149

Lang EK (1970) Superselective arterial catheterization of tumors of the urogenital tract: a modality used for perfusion with chemotherapeutic agents and infarction with radioactive pellets. J Urol 104:16–25

Lang EK, Nourse MH, Wishard WN, Mertz JH (1966) Accuracy of preoperative staging of bladder tumors by arteriography: a 5 year study. J Urol 95:363–368

Laux G, Cabanac U (1930) Artères iliaques. Anomalies. Arch Soc Sci Biol Montpellier 3 Rascicule

Ledwich E (1887) Absence of the internal iliac artery. J Med Dublin 83

Lepage T (1974) Embolisation en urologie. Medical dissertation, University of Paris

Levin DC, Stalano BS, Sceneider M, Becker A (1975) Complementary role of sonography and arteriography in management of uterine choriocarcinoma. AJR 125:462–468

Lindenbaum B, Sanders RJ, Steele G (1978) Persistant sciatic artery and sciatic artery aneurysm: a hazard in hip surgery. Clin Orthop J 132:68–70

Lipschutz BA (1978) A composite study of the hypogastric artery and its branches. Ann Surg 67:585–609

Louis R (1961a) Vascularisation artérielle de la vessie. Trav Lab Anat Marseille 19:45–66

Louis R (1961b) Vascularisation artérielle de la prostate. Trav Lab Anat Marseille 19:67–75

Louis R, Argencon C (1961) Contribution à l'étude de la vascularisation du rectum par l'artère hémorrhoïdale moyenne. Trav Lab Anat Marseille 19:77–89

Macarini N, Reggiani G, Scursatone M (1959) L'arteriografia della pathologica pelvica. Minerva Med 8:3601

Mannoni FX (1957) Vascularisation artérielle de la vessie. Medical dissertation, University of Bordeaux

Marchal G, Paleirac R, Colin R, Thevenet A (1953) La vascularisation artérielle du rectum. CR Assoc Anat (Paris) 11:276–283

Margolies MN, Ring EJ, Waltman AC, Kerr WS, Baum S (1972) Arteriography in the management of hemorrhage from pelvic fractures. N Engl J Med 287:317–321

Marley A, Schieino A (1964) Angiography in pelvic pathology: arteries, veines and lymphatics. Minerva Radiol 9:473–486

Marsault C, Le Guillou M, Bories J, Kuss R (1974) L'embolisation dans les cancers du rein: une aide dans le traitement des grosses tumeurs. Ann Radiol (Paris) 17/6:629–632

Marty F, Guignier M, Baudain P, Champetier M, Geindre M (1974) Intérêt de l'angiographie dans les complications hémorrhagiques des fractures du bassin. Ann Radiol (Paris) 17/6:633–637

Merland JJ, Bories J (1976) L'embolisation ou thrombose thérapeutique endoartérielle: une acquisition récente en radiologie vasculaire. A propos de 150 cas. Rev Med (Paris) 17:683–695

Merland JJ, Le Guillou M, Le Page T, Bories J, Kuss R (1974) Artériographie hypersélective et embolisation en pathologie génito-vésicale chez l'homme. Techniques-Résultats-Indications. Ann Radiol (Paris) 17:611–627

Miller FJ Jr, Mortel R, Mann WJ, Jahshan AR (1976) Selective arterial embolization for control of hemorrhage in pelvic malignancy: femoral and brachial catheters approaches. AJR 126/6:1028–1032

Mitchell ME, Waltman AC, Athanasoulis CA, Kerr WS, Dretler SP (1976) Control of massive prostatic bleeding with angiographic techniques. J Urol 115/6:692–695

Mitty HA, Baron MG, Jacobson JH (1968) Pelvic arteriovenous malformations. AJR 102/2:424–430

Neifeld JP, Doppman JL, Chretien PB (1975) Congenital pelvic arteriovenous fistulas: report of a case and review of the literature. J Urol 114/4:648–652

Newton TH (1963) The axillary artery approach to arteriography of the aorta and its branches. AJR 2:275–283

Nicholson RL, Patershank SP, Bnaradwaj BB (1977) Persistant primitive sciatic artery. Radiology 122/3:683–689

Nylander G, Petterson F, Swedenborg J (1978) Localized arterial occlusions in patients treated with pelvic field radiations for cancer. Cancer 41/6:2158–2161

Oka N, Sugiura N, Waswida W (1972) Roentgenological studies on the prostatic circulation. Nippon Hinyokika Gakkai Zasshi 63:229–234

Olcott C, Newton TH, Stoney RJ, Ehrenfeld WK (1976) Intra arterial embolization in the management of A.V.M. Surgery 89/1:3–12

Ollivier J (1969) Les lésions de l'artère hypogastrique et de ses branches dans les traumatismes du bassin. Mémoire CES Electroarad, University of Paris

Paster SB, Wanhouten FX, Douglass FA (1974) Percutaneous balloon catheterization: technique for control of arterial hemorrhage caused by pelvic trauma. JAMA 230:573–575

Paturet G (1958) Traité d'anatomie humaine. Masson, Paris

Penaud MG (1936) Recherches anatomiques sur les artères de la vessie. Medical dissertation, University of Bordeaux

Pereiras RV, Meier WL, Katz ER, Viamont EM (1977) Arteriographic embolization treatment for post prostatectomy hemorrhage. Urology 9/6:705–707

Perlberger RR (1977) Arteriographic localization and treatment of hemorrhages in pelvic fractures. Med J Geneeskd 1:9–11

Poirier P, Charpy A, Nicolas A (1914) Traité d'anatomie humaine. Masson, Paris

Reboul H (1953) Artériographie des membres et de l'aorte abdominale. Masson, Paris

Richelme H, Courbier R (1956) Valeur anastomotique des artères sacrées. Trav Lab Anat Marseille 16:49–54

Rinaldi I, Fitzer PM, Whitley DF, Peach WF Jr, Umstott CE, Graham WH, Winfrey EW (1976) Aneurysm of the inferior gluteal artery causing sciatic pain. Case report. J Neurosurg 44/1:100–104

Ring EJ, Athanasoulis C, Waltman AC, Margolies MN, Baum S (1973) Arteriographic management of hemorrhage following pelvic fracture. Radiology 109:65–70

Ring EJ, Athanasoulis C, Smith JC Jr, Baum S (1974) Angiography in pelvic trauma. Surg Gynecol Obstet 139:375–380

Sautot J, Mathon C, Duquesnel J (1970) Angiodysplasie avec fistule artério-veineuse du système hypogastrique droit. Lyon Chir 5:319–320

Schroeder J, Terwey B, Buar HJ, Gerhardt P (1978) Embolization treatment of traumatic pelvic hemorrages. Chirurg 49/5:286–289

Schwartz PE, Goldstein HM, Wallace S, Rutledge FN (1975) Control of arterial hemorrhage using percutaneous arterial catheter techniques in patients with gynecologic malignancies. Gynecol Oncol 3/4:276–288

Senior A (1925) An interpretation of the recorded arterial anomalies of the human pelvis and thigh. Am J Anat 36:46

Sheldon GF, Winestrock DP (1978) Hemorrhage from open pelvic fracture controlled intraoperatively with balloon catheter. J Trauma 18/1:68–70

Shiraishi T (1974) La valeur diagnostique de l'artériographie pelvienne dans les tumeurs de la vessie. Nippon Hinyokika Gakkai Zasshi 36/2:188–193

Sibuet J (1969) Contribution à l'étude de la circulation collatérale artérielle du petit bassin. Medical dissertation, University of Paris

Smith RS (1971) Pelvic arteriography in the differential diagnosis of pelvic mass. Am J Obstet Gynecol 11:952–958

Smith DC, Wyatt JF (1977) Embolization of the hypogastric arteries in the control of massive vaginal hemorrhage. Obstet Gynecol 49/3:317–322

Sutton D (1952) Placental and pelvic angiography by retrograde percutaneous injection of the femoral artery. Br J Radiol 25:320–325

Tage H, Thorkild M (1974) Control of life threatening vesical hemorrhage by unilateral hypogastric artery muscle embolization. J Urol 112:60–63

Takarashi M, Nagata I (1971) Angiography of trophoblastic tumors: correlation of pelvic angiography with direct fourfold magnification angiography of uterine specimen. AJR 112:779–787

Taylor DA, Macken KL, Weenemm RJ, Bachman AL (1965) A preliminary report of a new method for the staging of bladder carcinoma using a triple contrast technique. Br J Radiol 38:667–672

Tejmarova J (1972) Pelvic angiography in the diagnosis of urinary bladder tumors. Cesk Radiol 26:225–238

Testut L, Latarjet A (1949) Traité d'anatomie humaine. Doin, Paris

Thomas ML, Blakeney CG, Browse NL (1978) Arteriomegaly of persistent sciatic arteries. Radiology 128/1:55–56

Tokunaga T (1974) L'artériographie pelvienne dans les tumeurs de la vessie et de la prostate. Nippon Hinyokika Gakkai Zasshi 36/2:184–187

Tskanis P (1929) Les pédicules vasculaires de la vessie et son territoire chez l'homme. Medical dissertation, University of Paris

Villemin F, Rigaud A, Gouaze A (1952) Le tronc de l'artère hypogastrique. Variations en fonction du sexe. Un cas d'absence de ce tronc. Intérêt chirurgical. Sem Med 28:2–11

Vonwiller P (1929) Une anomalie artérielle rare: naissance de l'artère épigastrique à partir de l'artère hypogastrique. Ann Anat Pathol 6:1145–1150

Wenger JJ, Barth M, Tongio J, Bollack C, Warter P (1977) Radiological appearances of a pelvic schwannoma. J Radiol Electrol Med Nucl 58/6–7:475–8

Wheeler GW, Simmons CR (1973) Angiography in post-traumatic priapism. A case report. AJR 119/3:619–620

White RI, Strandberg JV, Gross GS, Barth KH (1977) Therapeutic embolization with long term occluding agents and their effects on embolized tissues. Radiology 125/3:677–687

Winterberger AR, Murphy GP (1974) Correlation of B scan ultrasonic laminography with bilateral selective hypogastric arteriography and lymphography in bladder tumors. Vasc Surg 8/3:169–176

Winterberger AR, Kenny GM, Choi SW (1972a) Correlation of selective arteriography in the staging of bladders tumors. Cancer 29:332–337

Winterberger AR, Jennings EC, Murphy GP (1972b) Arteriography in metastatic tumors to the bladder. J Urol 108:577–580

Winterberger AR, Wajsman Z, Nerrin C, Murphy GP (1978) Eight years of experience with preoperative angiographic and lymphographic staging of the bladder. J Urol 119/2:208–212

6 Subject Index